# the fastest
# diet

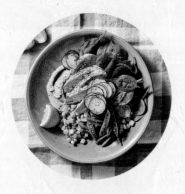

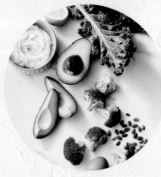

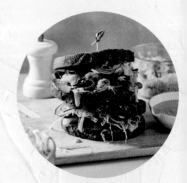

"I love that
you can't fail!
You really can't!"
**DORTE**

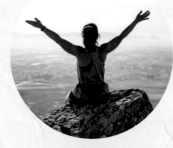

"It works, it's
not a huge effort
and it's easy to
keep it off"
**MARY**

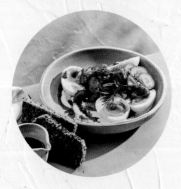

"I love that it's
not really a diet
but a way of life
that can adapt
to your needs"
**KELLIE**

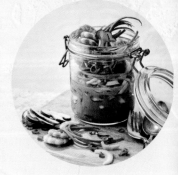

# the
# fastest
# diet

## The intermittent fasting formula *that will* supercharge your weight loss

**PROFESSOR KRISTA VARADY,
VICTORIA BLACK** *and* **GEN DAVIDSON**

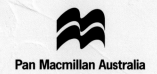

Pan Macmillan Australia

# Contents

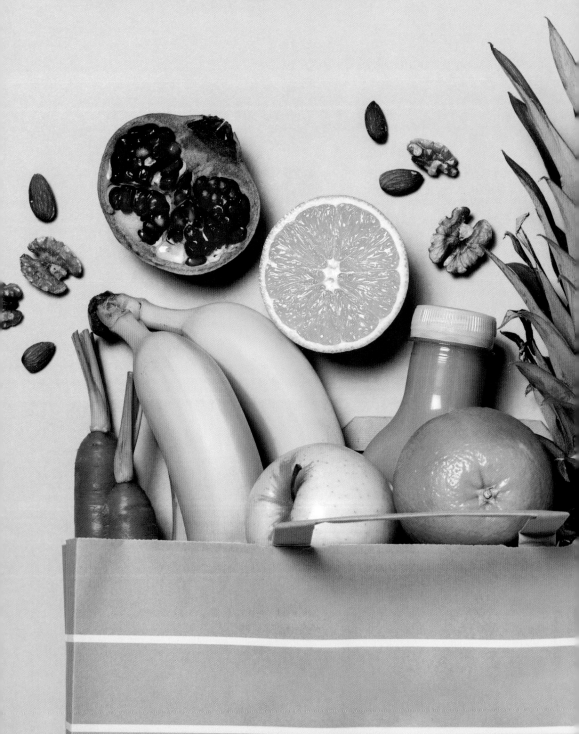

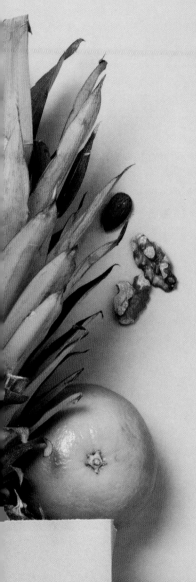

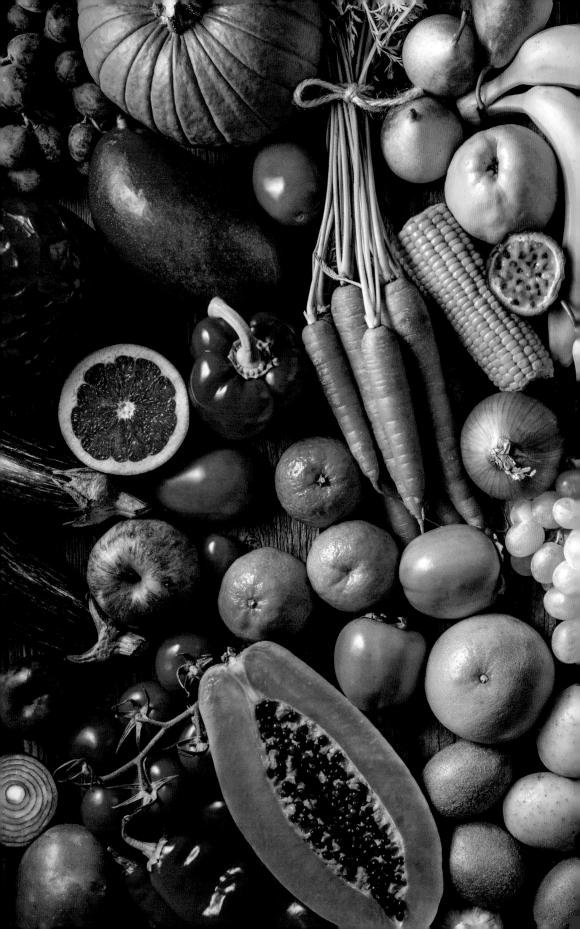

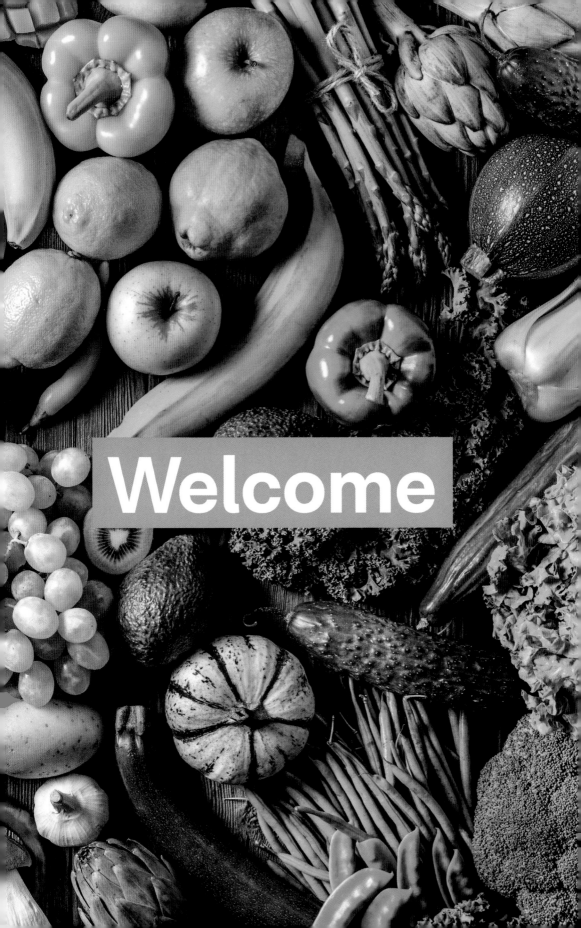

Welcome

# You're not just holding a book – you're holding the answer

If you're reading this, then you've been looking for 'that book' for some time, right? The one that will help you lose weight with ease and still enjoy all the food and drinks you love.

Well, give yourself a massive high-five because right here, right now, you haven't just started a book, you've started a healthier, happier life. This book really is the answer you've been looking for all this time and the diet struggle is over. For good. #winning

Those days of living on carrot sticks are well and truly gone and you're actually about to have a whole lot of fun on this diet – yes, fun. Those two words 'fun' and 'diet' can actually co-exist in a sentence because this really is a **fun diet**. Thanks to something called intermittent fasting (IF), you will lose weight, learn healthy habits and change your life. All good stuff – but you know what? You're still going to be able to enjoy life too, like eating out and getting social. #VerymuchWINNING

## Intermittent fasting – The Fastest Diet

What makes this book different from every other diet book? Because IF works. Oh, and because it's based on the very latest findings by world-leading fasting expert and our co-author, Dr Krista Varady from the University of Illinois, Chicago. Dr Krista has been the inspiration behind our revolutionary diet program ever since we met her at the Global Obesity Conference and heard about her extraordinary research. We decided then and there to take IF to the world and we have! Yet now she's had even more major breakthroughs and IF has reached a whole new level – especially combined with our own newest method: **supercharging** (more about that later).

> **IF isn't just a way of life - now it's actually and literally The Fastest Diet in the world and you're about to find out why - and how to do it for yourself!**

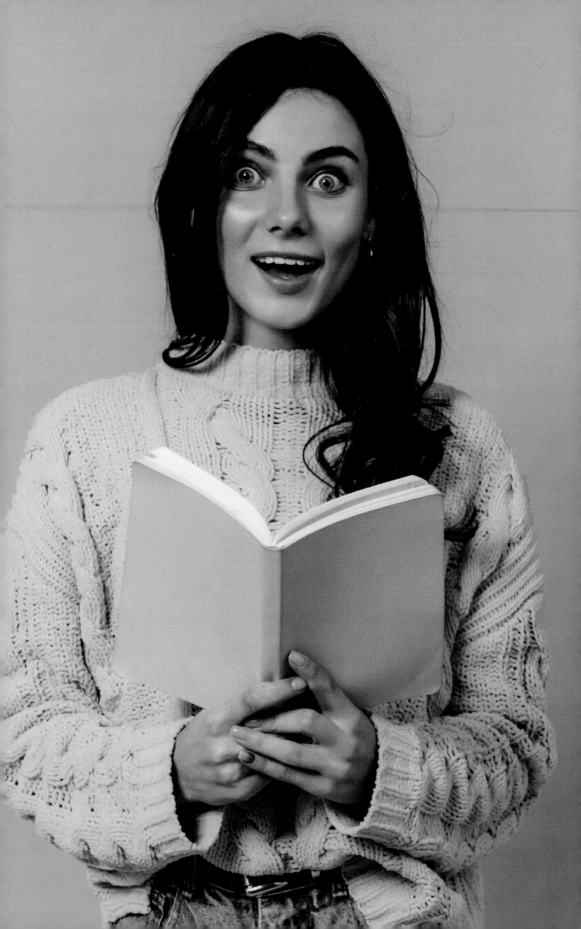

## So what makes intermittent fasting the answer?

- **Science says so.** And Dr Krista isn't alone in discovering this! Multiple groundbreaking scientific studies show that IF works because it is easy to stick to and it comes with a long list of whole-body benefits (like less inflammation, healthier guts and less belly fat). However, now there's even more exciting news – IF can reverse type 2 diabetes, plus a whole lot more! We can't wait to tell you more about Dr Krista's life-changing findings.

- **It's long-term by design.** IF is more like a lifestyle than a diet. We take you through several different methods that work IF into your daily routine. It's a way of eating that can chop and change depending on your goals and what life is demanding of you. This includes switching it up during holidays, for social events, during your hormonal cycles (for women) and even after you've hit your weight-loss goals. This makes maintenance easy and means that you reap the health benefits of fasting. For good.

- **It's super doable!** IF is really a part-time diet, which means it's mostly about when you eat. Of course what you eat and how much you eat can play a part too, but studies have shown that the scientific effect of delaying eating is the reason why IF works so well. That means no rigid rules, no strict meal planning and no saying goodbye to cheese and ice-cream forever. #totallyTOTALLYwinning

## Still, we know what you're thinking ... *but will intermittent fasting work for ME?*

IF works for just about anyone, as millions of advocates can testify to. (Did we mention it's the number-one diet in the world right now?) Tens of thousands of our readers and members have changed their lives with SuperFastDiet, and we're talking from personal experience as this all began because it worked for us in the first place.

Yes, we've stacked on weight in the past and tried all the diets and gym gizmos under the sun, only to fail. Yes, we've known the despair of thinking we could never feel like 'us' again and yes, we have suffered with health issues due to excess weight. Then along came IF, transforming our lives, giving us back our health, our confidence and our mojo, baby! We wanted to share that with as many people as we possibly could.

It just works! And we can't wait to show you the results of Dr Krista's latest groundbreaking scientific studies that show you why.

We'll also share the success stories of people who have lost weight with SuperFastDiet's part-day (16:8), 2-day (5:2), 3-day (4:3) and supercharging methods. They all did it their way to make it work for their lives, so reading their stories isn't just inspirational, you'll learn tips and tricks that you can use to make IF easily work for you, too. We'll also guide you by sharing best practices AND 'life' practices that render this part-time dieting lifestyle virtually unbreakable.

We totally get the mind games involved with trying to lose weight. Overcoming this was a huge part of our success so we've also included motivation and habit hacks to help you reach your goals and beyond.

Finally, and deliciously, there's the food! This book is packed full of amazing recipes, meal plans and food tips to help you cook and eat your way to weight-loss triumph. Our approach to IF is definitely from a food lover's perspective, so not only will you learn how to eat for nutrition and results, you'll be enjoying every mouthful along the way!

## The fastest diet – supercharging

Our three main methods of IF are literally 'fast' ways to lose weight at the best of times but this book also includes the **supercharging** method – a combo technique we've developed at SFD to up the fasting ante. Now, some of you keen beans will want to jump right into supercharging (and go for it, if that's you!). However, for those that need more of a roadmap, we've set up a guide for your first four weeks to help you learn about our three main methods first, then try supercharging.

## It's all about you

We put this book out into the world because we have exciting new findings to share from Dr Krista's research and we can't wait to tell you about supercharging! Plus, it's packed with everything else we wish we'd had to kick-start our journey: the ultimate guide, all the tips and tricks, the advice of others who've nailed this, awesome low-cal yet mouthwatering and nutritious food ... so yes, you'll learn about IF and how to use it to lose weight. But you'll also learn a lot about you.

There are to-do lists, reflections, mindset exercises, step-by-steps and activities that will help you discover what you need to succeed, how you want to live, what you love to eat and drink, what blocks you and what inspires you ... and ultimately what amazing results you're capable of!

The Fastest Diet isn't a quick fix, although we have seen results come quickly. It's a forever fix where we show you how to make IF the easiest, flexiest and life-proofiest way to the most fabulous you.

**This book is packed full of amazing recipes, meal plans and food tips to help you cook and eat your way to weight-loss triumph.**

## Girls (and boys!) just wanna have fun dieting – WHAAATTT?!

If there's one constant that's been true for us, it's that life should be fun. It should be sparkly! Bright! Colourful! Would you expect anything less from a friendship born in the 80s?

Back then, we both worked for an American weight-loss chain. If you're picturing tights, G-string leotards, fuzzy hair and a mish-mash of ALL the neon colours, you've got our looks just about right. We loved it and we felt genuinely excited to motivate women to find their best selves.

Unfortunately, the method was rather crazy. The gym was filled with wacky machines and our plates were filled with drab salads. We couldn't help but imagine there was a better way. Not just a set of exercises, magic machines or deprivation diets ... but something that was easy, effective and approachable. Something holistic that tackled multiple facets of the weight-loss challenge. We just didn't know what that was. So, on we went, bouncing around the 'figure-salons' (yes, they were actually called that) and doing our best to help women feel like they could reach the weight-loss stars on their StairMaster.

It was relatively easy for us to stay trim in those days. We had the time, motivation and resources. Then life happened. We had kids, built careers (Vic went into magazine publishing and marketing, while Gen set up a chain of gyms) – and worked hard at the heart-and-soul stuff of life. But the side-effect of that was stress, grown-up bills, school runs and 'seriously, is it Christmas already?' time-warps. Staying in shape while living this version of life wasn't as easy and our waistlines, arm-lines and thigh-lines slowly got out of control.

Seeing the numbers on the scales get higher and higher was one thing, but feeling so far away from our true selves was quite another. We couldn't wear the clothes we wanted to anymore, we had less energy, developed niggling health issues and felt frustrated and unhappy. We missed the former, vital versions of us and tried everything to get back to our glory days. There was the eggplant diet, lemon detox, the baby food diet, the Israeli Army Diet, the Vogue Wine and Egg Diet (fun but not very healthy – there was even a glass of wine with breakfast), and soooo many crazy cleanses. You name it, we tried it.

Through it all we stayed in touch – we still shared a passion for personal development and had a #dietfail confidant in each other. It was during one of these catchups in 2015 (over lunch, naturally) that got us on the road to SuperFastDiet.

## Finding the one

See, Gen had already started her fasting journey and turned up to lunch with a bangin' new bod! Ever the cheerleader, and genuinely shocked, Vic showered Gen with praise, excitement and a million questions. Namely: HOW?!

The elephant in the room (it definitely wasn't Gen) was the thought that maybe, just maybe, she had found 'THE answer'. The one we'd been looking for all these years. The one that actually worked!

'The one' was intermittent fasting (IF). Basically, IF is a way of short-term fasting, then feasting, that allows you to lose weight effectively, keep it off, and live an awesome life!

Inspired by Gen as living proof, and armed with all the research to back it up from Dr Krista and other world leaders in health (more about that soon), Vic gave it a go by trying the 2-day (5:2) and part-day (16:8) fasting methods. This meant either eating fewer calories on two out of seven days a week, or eating within eight hours a day. So basically, a part-time diet. This allows time for eating out and staying social – happy-hour drinks included. Vic ended up losing that stubborn 10 kg and we both regained our sparkle! But we never regained the weight.

This lit the fasting fire. It was the easy, effective and approachable diet we'd been looking for and we were itching to encourage as many women as we possibly could to give it a go, too. Lots of research, interviews with doctors, meetings with internationally renowned scientific researchers and vision boards later, we came up with what is now the SuperFastDiet program and phenomenon.

We were driven by the desire to approach weight loss in this new, holistic way. We'd lived through the struggle of other diets, so we knew this easy, flexible, mindset-focused and fun-driven way of life was a game changer.

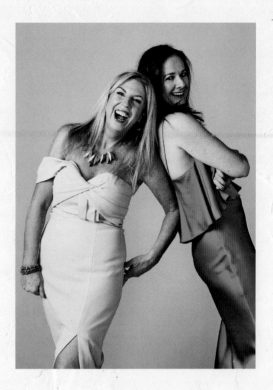

## Which brings us to...

SuperFastDiet! In 2018, we launched the SuperFastDiet program and online community, hoping to change as many lives as we could via our 2-day (5:2), 3-day (4:3) and part-day (16:8) methods. We developed meal plans and a library of recipes to inspire low-cal yet delicious culinary delights in the kitchen. We've built on a growing body of research that shows the myriad benefits of IF beyond weight loss, including the latest and most exciting findings from Dr Krista. Plus we've now developed supercharging, which is literally the fastest diet of all!

We now have a wealth of mindset and motivation to help keep you on track, plus we've written two bestselling books and created a mountain of content for our community. We're even award-winners, including the Australian Start-up Business of the Year in 2019! (Optus MyBusiness awards).

Most importantly, we have helped tens of thousands of REAL-LIFE SuperFasters who have gone on the SFD journey, lost the weight for good, gained confidence and found the best version of themselves, both inside and out. This is why we do it. We may have lost the fuzzy hair and neon lycra, but we're still those passionate coaches we were way back in the 80s, only this time we're showing you a far, far easier way to reclaim your body ... and your life.

We believe in IF. We believe in all the exciting research. We believe you can lose weight and socialise too on our part-time, unbreakable, fastest diet. We believe in this holistic, fun, easy way of life. We believe in you. And honey, you're about to believe in yourself, too!

# Gen's story

LOST 35 kg  Size 18 to size 8

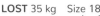

I am a fashionista, a Flake fanatic, a firm believer in the fiercely focused female – and I am forever grateful that I found fasting.

Like we said, it was easy for me to stay healthy while working in the salons and gyms – and let's face it – having all that energy in my twenties helped too. I've always truly believed in the potential that people carry within them to lose weight and live their best and healthiest lives. In my career, this meant coaching people through a plan of eating 1200 calories every day for months or burning off as many calories as they could with exercise to balance the energy in/energy out equation. However, it wasn't until I gained weight myself that I came to understand just how unattainable and difficult those methods were.

Like many women, I struggled to lose weight after I started a family in my thirties. By struggle, I mean STRUGGLE. I was on the weight-loss rollercoaster for almost 20 years trying desperately to stop gaining, but it kept creeping on. By the time I hit 50 I hardly recognised myself in the mirror, tipping the scales at 85 kg and pushing a size 18.

To make matters worse, I'd developed medical problems from carrying all that excess weight for so many years. I had sleep apnoea, high blood pressure and weak knees. I was also challenged mentally, feeling like I was a failure, especially since I used to coach people through this exact problem. It got to a point where I just gave up and resigned myself to an all-black wardrobe that hid everything about myself I loathed.

Then, I saw my brother-in-law Mark at a family gathering. He was dramatically trimmer since the time I'd seen him three months before, having lost 20 kg and he told me he was doing this new thing called intermittent fasting (IF). He was using the 2-day (5:2) method, which involved eating an average of 500 calories (for women) and 600 calories (for men) for two days, then eating normally the rest of the week. (Incidentally this original method was largely based on the scientific studies carried out by our co-author, Dr Krista Varady.)

What struck me was that Mark said it was the 'easiest thing' he'd done, and it was clearly working for him. Even though I was hesitant to put myself through the effort of another diet, I decided that I would try it for just one day. I prepped myself silly, making sure that I had as much food as I could fit into what sounded like a tiny allowance, telling myself that I could have pasta for breakfast tomorrow if I got through this one day (spoiler alert: I totally did).

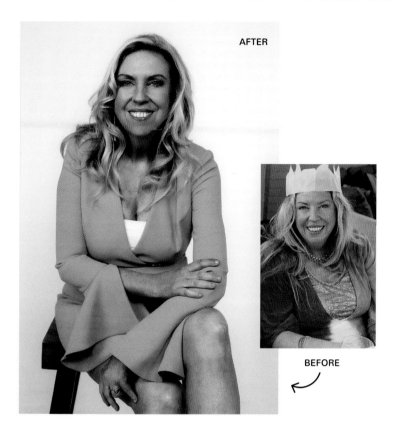

AFTER

BEFORE

With much shock and delight, I found that it was easy for me too. After that one successful day, then a normal day of eating (including breakfast pasta), I gave a second fast day a go. Again, to my surprise, I made it! By the end of my first fasting week I'd lost 2 kg.

It was a small win on the scales, but a huge win mentally. As the weeks went on, I found the best part about IF was that it was also flexible and forgiving. I didn't feel like I was missing out because I was still dining at restaurants, meeting friends for drinks and eating normally on holidays. And, when I had an inevitable slip-up, I just hit reset by swapping my fast day to the next day instead.

Eventually, I reached my goal of getting down to a size 8 and losing 35 kg. My health issues are all but gone and so is that dreary black wardrobe. Fasting brought me back to my sparkly self and I feel ah-mazing!

Gen

# Vic's story

**LOST** 10 kg    Size 14 to size 8–10

I am a self-confessed ice-cream-with-potato-chips type of girl and I love that intermittent fasting embraces such eccentricity! Anything goes on a part-time diet and that suits me down to a now smaller-sized tee.

My weight struggles have never been all that obvious as I've never been massively overweight. But here's the thing: body issues are all relative. In my youth – ahhh, youth – I was always fairly slim. (Although there was that one guy called Morris, a long blond-haired surfy type, who I thought was seriously spunky. Well, he announced that I would be quite pretty if I didn't have such a fat a$$! What a little sh1t!) When I graduated from university, I was actually really skinny. Although, granted, it was probably because I was on a European gap year, living on a $20-per-day budget. When I came home and started working with Gen at the weight-loss salons, I still found it easy to keep my weight under control.

That all changed when I started to pursue a career. My struggle with weight has largely been emotional and psychological. Shout-out to all the stress-eaters out there – I hear you!

Things got much harder after I had my first child, too. Balancing career and building a family is already challenging. Add to that the mental chatter that came with putting on 10 kg … Yep. Hard. Like Gen, I tried all the diets. My favourite was the Vogue Wine and Egg Diet, which didn't work but, hey, it was fun to try. Many of the diets yielded good results initially, but I'd always put the weight back on after the diet was 'over' and I got back to real life.

At my worst, I used to wake up and start my day with the thought, 'I'm fat'. Unsurprisingly, this set me on course for a horrid day of negative self-talk and internal stress. I'd go from snapping myself out of that damaging spell and trying to hang on to motivation all day, to coming home after a busy time at work and overeating because I was:

**a.** Stressed
**b.** Tired
**c.** Really, really hungry
**d.** All of the above

Then I'd wake up and do it all again. I was living a real-life (and very depressing) diet groundhog day.

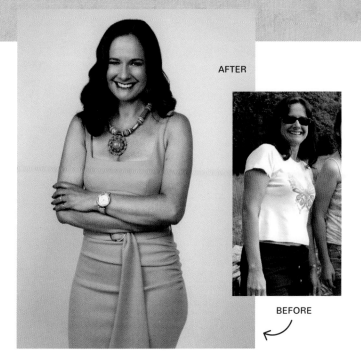

AFTER

BEFORE

It finally ended when I met Gen for lunch and she told me all about IF. She'd found her way back to her old self and, considering how amazing she looked and sounded, I decided I definitely needed to have what she was having.

I had 10 kg to lose, which may not sound like much, but that was what had a hold on me mentally. I was stuck for so long on the scales, I'd become stuck inside my head. When I finally lost it with IF, I felt like a totally new person and there wasn't a groundhog in sight.

The best bit was all the room that fasting allowed for imperfection. Life is imperfect, I'm imperfect, so for me all those other 24/7 diets were destined to fail when life needed to happen. With IF, you have 'on' and 'off' times. It really is part-time because you don't have to always be good. That makes it more of a lifestyle, which truly is unbreakable.

I could have my social life AND maintain my ideal weight! Literally having my cake and eating it too!

I feel like I've nailed it!

I feel so happy, energetic, confident, unstoppable ... strong and invincible in fact, and am SO unbelievably excited to help you feel that way too.

*Vic*

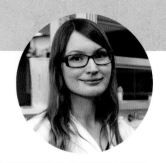

# Dr Krista's story

I am super passionate about fasting and finding the best ways to make it easy and effective for weight loss and wellness generally!

I've been studying IF for over 15 years as a professor of nutrition at the University of Illinois in Chicago. My very first study was small and only had about 20 participants. Back then, there really wasn't much research on IF. I actually thought it wouldn't work because people would find it too hard! So, the question we were testing back then was whether people could do it at all. We asked participants to try a regimen of 500 calories on one day, followed by no restriction on the following day, and alternating between those days for two months.

What we found (to my surprise) was that it worked really well! So well that, on average, people in that study lost between 4 and 13 kg. Since then, I've been involved in numerous research projects testing the effects of IF on weight loss, diabetes and fatty liver disease among other things.

My lab has also completed a 12-month study on time-restricted eating (or the part-day method), which is currently the longest study ever done. We share the details and results of these findings in this book but, in short, IF works extremely well for weight loss and people generally find it easy to stick to. A+!

The 'ease' of IF is a through-line that's been consistent in all my research. People get burned out from the effort of the 24/7 restriction that comes with traditional dieting. IF is an alternative that allows for much more freedom, and people like that.

They say that the most effective diet is the one you can stick to, and our studies show just that! Personally, I find it much easier than most other diets as it allows me to eat freely on non-fast days. I love that it can be simple – as a working mother of two, that's important.

On a personal level, I first tried alternate-day fasting after giving birth to my son. I desperately wanted to lose the 6.8 kg of baby weight that my body refused to shed. I tried daily calorie restriction first (which is kind of embarrassing since I am an IF researcher!), but I soon realised this was a mistake. I found it too hard to vigilantly monitor all of my calorie intake all the time. I had to record every meal, snack and drink on an app, every single day. It was way too tedious and I quit the diet within a week.

Then I switched to alternate-day fasting. I know I'm an expert but, in all honesty, I think I was worried that IF would be too intense while caring for a newborn baby. I thought that consuming only 500 calories every other day postpartum would lead me to feel even more exhausted and irritable. But boy, was I wrong. After a week of alternate-day fasting, my energy and mood improved considerably. In addition, I started losing about half a kilogram per week. It was terrific! I continued this fasting regimen until I reached my goal weight, which took about 12 weeks.

I still use IF as a tool for weight maintenance with the part-time method on weekdays. For me, this just means having dinner before 6–6:30 pm, then eating at around 10 or 11 am the following morning and fasting (mostly in my sleep – bonus!) in the hours between. I only do this on weekdays because I like to be able to eat socially on weekends and this works perfectly for me. We've also found in our studies that the part-time method still produces weight loss even if you don't count calories, so that's exactly what I do.

I also regularly use alternate-day fasting after the holidays each year. Like many of us, I find that I gain a few kilos after weeks of cocktail parties, dinners and other food-centred celebrations. So rather than missing out, I let myself celebrate, then course-correct in early January by incorporating four fast days into my week. I find that allows me to shed those extra holiday kilos and get back into my healthy habits after a few weeks.

Recently, I've discovered that fasting also helps me to control my ulcerative colitis. Colitis is a form of inflammatory bowel disease that can make it very painful to digest food. I've found that fasting is extremely helpful when I am experiencing a flare-up. Whenever I feel a flare coming on, I go on a water fast for a few days and this helps my symptoms subside almost right away.

In my experience and research, IF has proven to be effective for weight loss and can help treat (or even reverse) some major health issues. I personally love the flexibility of the diet and the immediate results I see every time I use it!

I'm so happy to share scientific findings that enable people to understand the benefits of IF and empower them with information they can use to drastically improve their health.

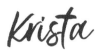

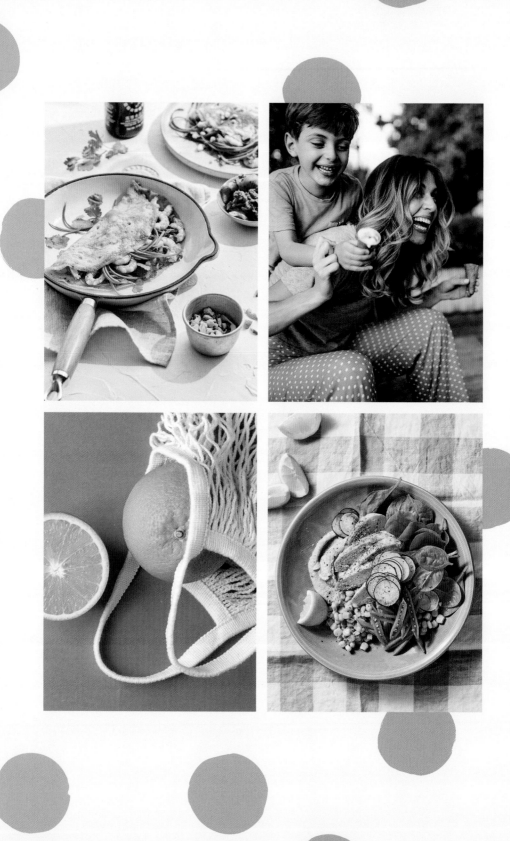

CHAPTER

1

# It's not really a diet, it's just ... life

# Why cavemen and women were onto something

As much as we'd love to take credit for inventing intermittent fasting (IF), we can't. It's actually as old as the hills – well, the cave-dwellers in them at any rate. Fasting has been around since Ms Trog accidentally dropped a hunk of meat into the fire and the practice of eating after a good hunting/gathering expedition is firmly embedded in our DNA.

Our bodies were trained for tens of thousands of years to adjust to periods of feasting when we found food, and periods of fasting when we had to sit around and draw paintings on the wall while we went without. We're built to feast and we're built to fast. It was quite literally just 'life' for the Trog family.

It's an ancient religious practice, too. Many of the world's oldest religions have observed (or still observe) the practice of fasting for spiritual reasons. If you grew up Catholic like Gen, you might remember those tummy rumbles before Mass or during Lent.

Fast forward to the present day. Many modern humans can eat whatever, whenever, thanks to refrigeration, supermarkets and restaurants. Gone are the days when you had to pick up your club and brave the unknowns of the scary jungle. These days our scary jungles consist of crowded carparks and neon-lit supermarkets, with everything your taste buds could possibly want, tantalisingly on display. You don't even have to brave the crowds, in fact. You can choose not to leave the couch at all and have a full meal delivered straight to your door. This means we can eat all ... the ... time. And many people do (us included, once upon a time).

The downside to all that ease of access is how easily it can lead to weight gain and the issues that come with it. The latest data from the Australian Bureau of Statistics (ABS) show that 67 per cent of adults are overweight or obese. Our ancestors may well have battled for their mammoth meal but at least they didn't have to battle obesity. There is good news for us modern humans, however, because we don't have to reinvent the diet wheel. We can simply replicate the Trogs' fast/feast lifestyle with IF.

## Um, so what actually *is* intermittent fasting?

Scientifically, the definition of IF is exactly as it sounds: intermittent periods of eating, interspersed with intermittent periods of not eating, or eating less. It's a behavioural approach to weight loss that works with the idea of 'delaying' food consumption rather than 'denying' it. In a nutshell, it is essentially a 'reward cycle' of eating (we told you it was fun – who doesn't love being rewarded?!).

For example, you might skip a meal or reduce calorie consumption for a while, but then you can fully enjoy a well-earned, hearty meal as your reward. Normal eating – delayed. Compare this with traditional calorie restriction diets when you're on a set number of calories for an extended period with no big pay-off rewards in sight. Normal eating – denied. Totally different mindset, right?

I have been with SuperFastDiet for over two years and have lost 20 kg, which I have maintained within a 2 kg range. Normally, when on a 'diet' I would regain all of the kilos along with a few extras as well. A conventional diet has a beginning and an end, but SFD is a lifestyle and you live it each day, which is the major difference. Another important thing to me is the SFD community itself, something that has always been a missing factor in my life. If I'm having a bad day, I just reach out and someone will be there to support me, as we are all on the same journey and are here to help each other. For anybody who has been on the diet treadmill like I have been, all I can say is give SFD a try. It worked for me and I was 60 when I began my journey.

**DONNA BLACK**

This 'reward yourself' point of difference is one of the keys to fasting success. It's much easier to stick to the diet because you regularly get to 'break' it when you end your fast, so it doesn't really seem like a diet at all. It's almost like you're cheating – even though you're not. (Although it does feel a bit naughty. Which we like.)

There are also health benefits to delaying eating, as your body actually gets to hop into a 'fasted' state. Think of IF like a boogie-nights dancefloor. You may well be a dancing queen, shaking your booty with the best of them, but sooner or later you literally need to cool your heels and take a break. Your body is the same. You could eat whatever you like at all times, but to achieve optimum health and weight, your body actually needs a break from eating so it's rested and ready to chow down in funky food town.

*Decide which days to fast in advance & plan according to your actual week – simple as that!*

## The flexy factor

IF is an umbrella term for a whole bunch of different methods or approaches. In the health-o-sphere, there are lots of terms to describe fasting. You might recognise 'The Warrior Diet' (eating for only four hours a day), 'OMAD' or 'One Meal a Day', or 'The 24-hour Fast', which is pretty much the same as OMAD. We've tried them all and narrowed our favourite methods to start with down to the 2-day (5:2), 3-day (4:3), part-day (16:8) and now 'supercharging' (more on that exciting new method in a sec!) as these are the ones that we've found the cinchiest to maintain.

The flexy factor comes into play with all of our methods. If you choose the 2-day, 3-day or supercharge methods, you can decide which days to fast in advance. A nice hack is to plan your fasting week according to your actual week. So, if you know you have something social scheduled for what is usually a fast day, you just move it to another day so you can go out and enjoy. Note: if you change your mind at the last minute because your BFF brought over a pizza, that's okay too. You can just move the fast day again. #winningwithcheeseontop

If you choose the part-day method, you're allowed to have an eating 'window' of about eight hours each day. Your chosen window can be anytime you like. If you're a big-time breakfast lover, you can shift your window and have an early dinner instead. If you're happy to skip breakfast, it's really just a normal day's eating otherwise. **Plenty of our members have lost significant amounts of weight simply by becoming 'breakfast-skippers'.**

**And ...** You can also change your method if you feel like you want to amp it up after reaching a goal.

**And ...** You can take it to the next level with a 'clean fast' or make it foolproof with a 'dirty fast' (more on that cheeky practice on page 57).

**And ...** You can also hit reset after you've overindulged/been on holidays/had a huge social weekend by supercharging.

In fact, there are so many IF tools you can pack in your kit, you'll feel like a superhero with an invisible fasting utility belt at your fingertips. It's not a static, unchangeable boring old diet with one set of rules. It's an adaptable way of eating that gives you diet superpowers you can access at any given time. #flexyfactor

I've been doing the SFD for six months now and have lost 7.8 kg. I've been a bit relaxed the last month as I had a house guest for two weeks – a little takeaway here, a little snacking there – and I still lost 2 kg ... I've needed to have a bra hook extender with my bras for years ... I have been able to take it out and am now on the last row of three hooks! I can also wear rings that I haven't been able to fit on my fingers for a very long time!

NICOLE HAND

## Intermittent fasting is a whole-body experience!

Prior to Dr Krista's latest research, this is everything we knew about the health benefits of fasting:

**Fasting is gutsy, in that it's good for your guts.** A 2020 study found that the diversity of the gut microbiome increased by 31 per cent in participants who fasted, compared to those that didn't. 'Um ... what's a microbiome?' we hear you ask. It's a clever community of microorganisms believed to be key for gut health.

**Fasting also increases 'good' cholesterol.** A 2020 study linked this increased microbiome richness with an increase in HDL cholesterol – that's the 'good' cholesterol that helps your body get rid of 'bad' cholesterol that can lead to heart disease and stroke.

**It can improve sleep apnoea.** A 2020 study on the effects of fasting on quality of sleep reported a decrease in sleep apnoea. Gen is real-life proof of this, no longer needing a machine or having to spend the night in the spare room! Participants in this study also reported no disruption to sleep patterns while they were fasting.

**Belly fat decreases.** Hooray! Multiple studies found a reduction in waist circumference in fasting groups, with one study reporting a median decrease of 4.6 cm after 90 days. Belly fat can be dangerous because it surrounds internal organs and can lead to health issues.

**It may help prevent cancer.** Multiple studies conducted since 2020 report a decrease in the hormone 'insulin-like growth factor' (IGF-1). In 2020, a study found that, in excess, IGF-1 may be associated with an increased risk of several cancers, including melanoma, thyroid cancer and bone marrow cancer.

**It may improve quality of life.** A three-month study published in 2022 had participants report a statistically significant improvement in quality of life. This was measured by questionnaires, including the World Health Organization standards, which tracked general mood, vitality, social functioning, mental health, emotional wellbeing and more. #happinessdiet

**It may increase energy.** The same 2022 study also found statistically significant reductions in physical and mental fatigue after three months. #energisingdiet

**It may improve brain function.** Researchers found that fasting can give your brain a boost by increasing the chemical 'brain-derived neurotrophic factor' (BDNF) that improves the connection between brain cells, hence improving brain function. #smartypantsdiet

**It may decrease blood pressure.** Multiple studies reported a decrease in blood pressure of between 3 and 11 per cent as a result of IF.

**It may improve mood and reduce anxiety and depression.** A review of studies that looked at the mental health effects of IF found that it effectively improved mood. Improvements in anxiety levels and depression in participants who fasted was also reported.

**There *will* be weight loss.** A scientific review of the part-day method reported that the most common finding in these studies was a decrease in body weight. Multiple studies also reported a decrease in body fat percentage and Body Mass Index (BMI). #weightloss=fact

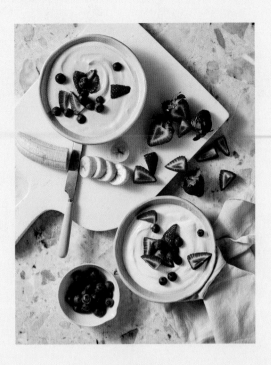

# Drum roll, please ...

## DR KRISTA'S LATEST FINDINGS!

As if this wasn't all enough, Dr Krista has made even more incredible scientific discoveries in her latest research, as revealed in Chapter 2, although, spoiler alert: there are not one, not two, but four eureka moments to share!

Nearly five years on from joining the wonderful SFD program, I still give thanks to Vic and Gen every day. Last week I went shopping for an outfit for my son's wedding ... It is a size EIGHT, before SFD I wore a size 18. Thank you.

SUE YOUNG

## Stickier than a sticky date

Let's face it, the most effective diet is the one that you can actually stick to. By far the best thing about IF is that it does stick because it truly is a lifestyle. We stuck to it, countless SuperFasters stuck to it and multiple scientific studies prove that it's realistic and feasible as a long-term solution to weight loss.

Why? Well, it's like the couple in your favourite rom-com: ending up together is always on the cards. When it comes to fasting, feasting is always on the cards too. Or at least it will be, very soon. It's only a matter of time until you and your fave foods are blissfully reunited once more.

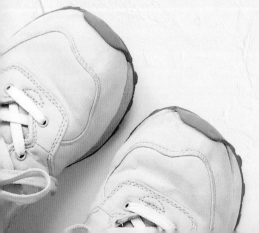

I have had some very big wins since joining SFD September 2021. In total I have lost nearly 15 kg but the biggest win for me was finding my tribe and, with their support, gaining control over how I feel, how I look and who I am. It is truly so doable and unbreakable. My body shape, fitness and control over cravings are just some of the spin-offs. It is holistic, not just a weight-loss program, and that is what makes it such a success.

**ANNETTE TWITE**

## The methods

Starting an IF program is different from starting other diets. This time, it's personal.

Choosing how you want to fast is completely up to you. In the words of Fleetwood Mac, you can go your own way and that's one of the reasons it works so well. Your lifestyle is the key determining factor, so choosing your method is really an exercise in you doing you.

As you read through the next section, keep these personal preferences in mind, including:

- When do you like to eat? If you're a bit meh about eating breakfast, that's about to become an advantage!
- When are you most social? Are you a bruncher, luncher, a diner or a cheese and winer?
- Do you have some days that could easily work as fast days as par for the course? Long work shifts? Travel times? Super busy days of the week? This becomes less important as you get used to fasting, but at the beginning it can be helpful if your first few fast days are filled with distractions like, you know, life.
- On the flip side, if you feel like a fast day will be easier if you're not busy and able to focus on your eating plan, take that approach instead.
- Kids, work, study, travel and special occasions are also worth considering, especially if they have a big impact on your schedule.

How you fast is as individual as you. Remember: you are now your very own weight-loss coach. And you make the rules.

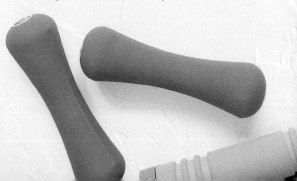

## THE 3-DAY METHOD

The 3-day method is based on a weekly timing schedule where you eat normally for four days and restrict your calories the other three. Ideally, these days are alternated.

On fast days, the average woman would consume up to 1000 calories and the average man 1200 calories. On regular days the average woman would consume up to 2000 calories and the average man 2400 calories. Yep, it's basically half the calories on fast days. Simple really. Your Total Daily Energy Expenditure (TDEE) is a calculation that will give you a more accurate personal recommendation. See more about this on page 59, or go to https://superfastdiet.com/what-is-tdee/

### WHO WILL LOVE IT?

The 3-day method works well for people that like fast days, but prefer more calories.

### 1000-CALORIE FAST DAY EXAMPLE

**Breakfast:** 60 g (¼ cup) Greek-style yoghurt with 6 strawberries and ¼ cup blueberries (145 calories). Small banana for a **mid-morning snack** (90 calories). A large multi-grain bread roll, a slice of low-calorie cheddar cheese, one sliced tomato, two slices sandwich ham for **lunch** (360 calories). Ten almonds plus tea/coffee with milk in the **afternoon** (93 calories). Grilled salmon with steamed vegies for **dinner** (322 calories). A bowl of diet jelly and a cup of herbal/fruit tea **before sleep** (7 calories) and waking up to a normal non-fast day tomorrow!

## THE 2-DAY METHOD

The 2-day method uses the same weekly timing, except you pick any two days of the week to fast. On the other five days, you eat your regular number of calories.

For the average woman, that's 500 calories on a fast day and 2000 on a regular day. For the average man, that's 600 calories on a fast day and 2400 on a regular day. That's basically a quarter of the calories on fast days, and again, you'll need to calculate your TDEE to get the right numbers for you. See more about this on page 59, or go to https://superfastdiet.com/what-is-tdee/

If 500 calories sounds like nothing, it's because it's a lot less food than most people are used to, but you'd be surprised at how much you can eat with a bit of planning. And don't forget, when you're on a fast day, you'll be able to eat much more tomorrow! Just the thought that you can have pretty much whatever you want tomorrow keeps you going!

### WHO WILL LOVE IT?

The 2-day method is great for people who want to get their fasting for the whole week done in two days and enjoy the rest of the week eating normally.

### 500-CALORIES FAST DAY EXAMPLE

**Wake up** with a cup of black coffee (or you can add a dash of milk) and eat 50 g Greek-style yoghurt with 100 g blueberries **mid-morning** (138 calories). Mountain-bread wrap with sliced turkey and lots of green salad and cherry tomatoes for **lunch** (150 calories). A carrot and a celery stick, cut into strips for an **afternoon snack** (34 calories). Stir-fry lamb with Mongolian sauce and Asian vegies for **dinner** (170 calories). Herbal tea or black tea with a dash of milk **before sleep** and waking up to a normal non-fast day menu!

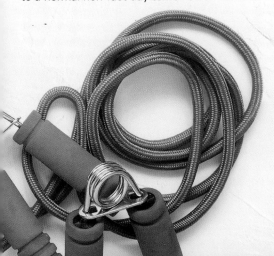

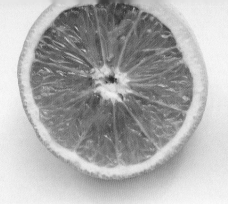
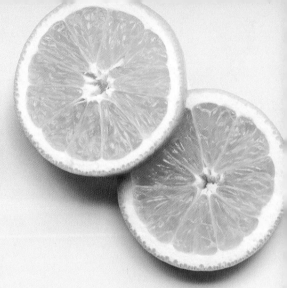

## THE PART-DAY METHOD

The part-day method of IF involves reducing the time you eat each day to eight hours. This is what we'll call your 'eating window'. Part-day fasting can be as simple as skipping breakfast and not snacking after dinner, or eating breakfast and having an early dinner in the evening.

A shorter eating window will naturally mean less calorie consumption for most people anyway, but we encourage calorie consumption of 1600 for the average woman and 1920 calories on average for men. This is about 20 per cent less than the average TDEE. See more about this on page 59, or go to https://superfastdiet.com/what-is-tdee/

### WHO WILL LOVE IT?

Part-day is best suited for people that don't want to feel like they're on a diet. There's a little effort at the start or end of the day when you're delaying food – but that's a lot less than 24/7 calorie counting or restriction. Especially if you take the eight hours you spend sleeping into account ... you're already halfway there!

### PART-DAY EXAMPLE

**Wake up** at 7 am, black coffee, tea and water until 1 pm when the eating window opens. Chicken, orange and spice-roasted chickpea salad for **lunch**. Popcorn **snack**. Mushroom stroganoff with parmesan for **dinner** at 7 pm followed by a **dessert** of low-calorie salted caramel parfait finished before the eating window closes at 9 pm. Have herbal tea to wind down **before sleeping** through most of your fasting window.

## Enter the SFD supercharging method

The SFD supercharging method of IF came about quite by accident. We got so in the habit of swapping the other three methods around, part-day kind of just meshed with 2-day or 3-day. The results were so much faster when we stuck to an eight-hour eating window regardless of what other method we were using we started calling it 'supercharging'. Then we mentioned it to our members who took to it like a credit card to a Black Friday sale – and the charging was on! It works so well, it's one of the main reasons we wrote this book with Dr Krista because SFD isn't just a fasting diet now, it's **The Fastest Diet**. See you on the (going) down low, unwanted kilos!

### HERE'S HOW IT WORKS

Supercharging uses the part-day principle of the eight-hour eating window to maximise the benefits of the 2-day or 3-day methods. Yep, it's basically a genius combo.

It can be used as the method you choose to lose and maintain weight for an extended period, or it can be a tool that you use to boost weight loss at any given time.

### WHO WILL LOVE IT?

Anyone who wants to maximise their weight loss with IF. Anyone who's been overindulging and needs a quick win. #postholiday-reset

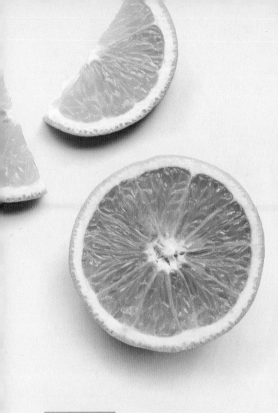

I joined SFD in July 2021 weighing in at 100.6 kg, the heaviest I had ever been. I set myself a target of losing 15 kg, doing the 2-day (5:2) method. Twelve months later, I weighed in at 65 kg! I dropped from a size 20 to size 12. My cholesterol is back in the normal range and so is my BMI. I walk nearly every day now. It sounds strange but at the age of 60, thanks to SFD, I have finally learned moderation in food, alcohol and treats. I continued to have wine and chocolate throughout my journey but I now understand what an appropriate portion is. I've been maintaining my new weight for four months now. I love that I can still eat all the foods I enjoy, and that weight gained on holidays is no longer permanent! Thank you, Vic and Gen, for introducing us to this doable, enjoyable, transformative way of life.

**ELIZABETH HOFFMAN**

Now, if you're experiencing a little information overload at this point remember: IF is super flexy. None of these options have to be forever. In fact, it's quite common for people to swap methods around as they reach new goals, or as their body becomes more accustomed to fasting. In Chapter 3, we give you a four-week road map that tells you exactly how to get started in a way that gives you a taste of all the methods, eases you into supercharging and leads you to awesome initial results!

If you're a bit overwhelmed by the food, calorie and nutrition side of things too, we get it. No one has the time to become a nutritionist, health expert and chef on top of normal life, and you won't have to be.

The whole point is to lose weight and get healthy *easily*. Our approach to the techy stuff and info is more to explain how it 'should' work in a perfect world, then show you how to apply it in the real world.

Remember the superhero utility belt? Sometimes, especially in the beginning, you'll need to use these superpowers and tools while you find your fasting feet. Even after you've done IF for a while, you might need them to rebound from a setback or get through a period of busyness, holidays or low motivation. The fact is, whenever you need them, they're right there, ready to save the day.

*No one has the time to become a nutritionist, health expert and chef on top of normal life, and you won't have to be.*

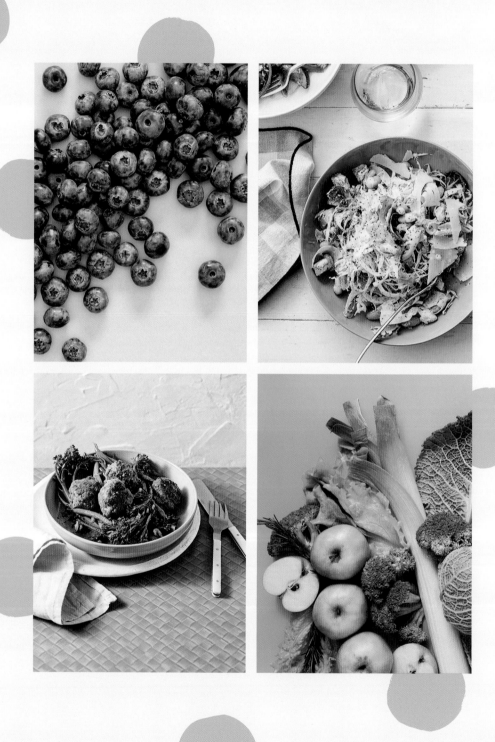

CHAPTER

2

# Your body actually *is* a wonderland

# Your amazing bodily self

Your body is Attenborough-level amazing, even though you want to change it. It is incredible. Right now. Think about it: every ancestor that came before you – all the way back to when we were living Trog-style and beyond – contributed to the intricately complex, seemingly miraculous design that is you.

Some days, when you're on the couch face-first into a family pack of cheesy snacks, it might not feel like you're a scientific wonder/ Michelangelo-level work of art, but you are!

There's a whole world of scientific, incredulous stuff going on every second of your existence that you're likely largely unaware of: little cells carrying stuff around your micro-universe; big organs calling the shots to keep you at maximum health as they perform a zillion miniature tasks each day. Chemistry, biology, psychology, neurology – your body actually is a wonderland!

It's just a wonder we don't come with instructions. Luckily for us, our clever, bodily selves do the 'other' thinking for us so we can remain blissfully unaware as we go about the business of sleeping/working/occasional couch-snack-bingeing etc. Still, it's helpful that scientists do their best to understand what's going on in there. By knowing what those industrious body bits and bobs are up to, we can better understand why we need to do certain things like IF, and help our bodies to stay in tip-top shape.

*Autophagy is like the Marie Kondo of our cells, deciding what needs to be thrown away.*

## Hungry eyes: the science of eating

Can you believe that eating is more than just sitting at a table, tasting delicious food and pondering seconds?!

To our body, eating is a huge deal. Okay, to our minds, too. But parts of our insides react like elves in Santa's factory preparing for Christmas at the prospect of eating. Think about the way you salivate over the thought of a meal, or how your stomach grumbles at lunchtime. These are all signs that our body is busily getting ready to metabolise (aka deconstruct) food.

The whole point of eating, from our body's biological point of view, is to break food down into bits that it can use as fuel to build, maintain and repair cells. The 'breakdown' of food happens in our digestive system. It starts in our mouth with chewing and saliva and ends ... er, flushed away. A lot of elf-work goes on in between as our stomach and intestines, pancreas and liver work hard to break food down and make their deliveries to the rest of the body.

Here's a breakdown of the food breakdown:

**carbohydrates** turn into **glucose;**

**protein** to **amino acids; and**

**fats** into **fatty acids.**

(Don't worry, we'll get into more detail about how that translates to what you should actually put on your plate in Chapter 4.)

When our body is doing all this, we're in a 'fed' state, which is good because we need these nutrients and energy for our body to work. When we're done processing that food – and it usually takes about five to six hours – we enter a 'fasted' state when our body undergoes a bunch of other processes and mechanisms that are just as important.

An example is something called 'autophagy', the Marie Kondo of our cells. All the chemical reactions that take place can sometimes leave a little mess. Autophagy, like Marie, comes in and decides what is useful to the cell for recycling and what needs to be thrown away. Does it spark digestive joy? No? Then out she goes! The result is a super-schmick cell that functions to organised perfection! The catch is that autophagy can only take place when we're in a fasted state. Think of it this way – would Marie come and declutter with a constant stream of new things coming through the door and filling up the house? No. Autophagy only gets to work when nothing new is coming through your digestive door, aka when you're in a fasting state.

The body works best when it gets the chance to be 'fed' and 'fasted'. Biological processes that happen when we are fed tend to only happen when we are fed. Biological processes that happen when we fast tend to only happen when we fast. If one happens for too long (for most people this is feeding), those processes become strained or get in the way of others happening at all. This can lead to weight gain and poor health. The bottom line? Your body loves fasting just as much as it loves feeding. #digestivejoysparked

## The key to unlocking fat stores

If we could change the way our body worked, the first thing we'd likely do is allow it to thrive on a diet of cheese, cocktails and cake. The second thing we'd do is to turn on fat-burning 24/7. Until we figure out a way to do that, we'll just have to work with what we've got, and the best way to do it is with fasting.

The fat on our body isn't there just to make us feel bad. It's pretty crucial for a lot of things, like vitamin absorption, insulation, physically protecting organs and storing backup energy. Ms Trog and her tribe relied on these fat energy stores to get them through periods of food scarcity when the mammoth were nowhere to be found. In the age of supermarket-shopping ease, many of us have an excess of fat that we don't really need. Yep, we are literally shopping at the fat stores these days. (Sorry, that joke was just sitting there waiting to be made.)

When it comes to burning energy, the body likes to take the path of least resistance. Nutritionally, this means using carbohydrates (as glucose) first, fat next and protein last. If we eat more carbohydrates than we use, we store it as glycogen in the liver and muscles where it can easily be turned into glucose for energy.

Sounds fine in theory, only we tend to fill up those glycogen stores pretty fast and they often don't get used, resulting in any excess carbohydrates getting converted into fat and stored away. Our body will never skip those steps and burn fat if we're always feeding. It's as futile as wishing cheese, cocktails and cake had zero calories. Ain't gonna happen!

One reason is that when we eat, our pancreas gets a ping to produce insulin. Insulin is important as it helps absorb sugar from our blood and tells the body to convert it into glycogen and body fat as stored energy. In other words, insulin tells the body

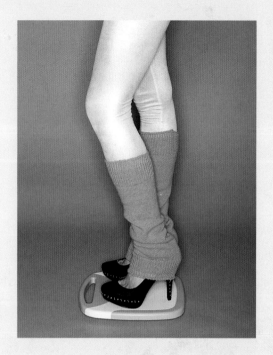

## If we need fat, why is obesity an issue?

Body fat is stored in special 'adipose tissues' and just like you, they have limited wardrobe space. Once these adipose tissues are at capacity, our body stores fat in other places that aren't designed to keep it. This compromises the function of these organs and the cells inside it because, put simply, the fat is in the way. If all that extra clothing has filled the spare room and started filling other parts of the house, your day-to-day routine gets disrupted. A healthy fat cell can be 90 per cent fat and function well; a liver cell filled with any more than 20 per cent fat is sick.

that there's food available and that it needs to be stowed. If we're continually feeding our body and producing insulin, we don't allow it to process that stored-away fat.

So how do we unlock fat stores? Simple: we go through the windows! Having clear eating and not-eating windows (fasting) puts the body into fat-burning mode. When we're fasting, insulin isn't released and other hormones start using fat rather than storing it. Fasting allows our body to run on the fat that we already have because we've stopped producing more.

It's kind of like how you forget about all the clothes that get pushed deeper into your bulging wardrobe as you fill it with new ones. Over time, your wardrobe will start to overflow – which sounds good because hey, fashion – but in reality, you've got a whole bunch of outfits you don't wear but you never clean it out because you're always shopping, adding more. You're never going to burn the body fat you have stored unless you stop adding more either. Fat/fashion fact.

## You vs your bodily self

At this point, formal introductions may be in order. You, meet your bodily self. Your bodily self, meet you. As explored earlier, you actually have two 'thinking' processes going on inside your body/brain, and you're not always on the same page. In fact, you can see/experience things quite differently and the sooner you can understand those differences, the faster you can work better together. Because, here's the thing: you're both right. And we all love to be right. But when it comes to biology, you kind of have to listen to your body too.

In Chapter 4, we get into the nitty gritty of food and calories. Understanding how this works on a body level will help you make the most of IF by making smarter food choices.

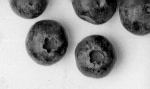

| The thing | What you think it is | What your bodily self thinks it is |
|---|---|---|
| **Food** | A necessary part of life that satisfies taste and hunger. | Energy and nutrients that fuel all the mechanisms that keep you alive. |
| **Eating** | An experience you look forward to and relish when it's delicious. | The ignition of processes that make up digestion. |
| **Fasting** | Starving. | Time for digestive mechanisms to take a break and for the cleaning and repair mechanisms to kick in. |
| **Calories** | Numbers that add up to how much food you can eat in a day. Or on the back of a label, a sign of whether food is naughty or nice – e.g. 65 calories from a boiled egg = nice snack that won't take too many calories away from my allowance. | The amount of energy you can get from food to use as fuel – e.g. after you break the egg down, you'll have 65 calories to use as fuel in your body. |
| **Fat** | The thing you don't want to be, but also the thing that usually tastes so damn good. It's complicated. | Backup energy. Also, fat cells keep us warm and protected. We need fat, but not too much. It's complicated. |
| **Carbohydrates** | The sugary, bready, pasta, rice stuff that you constantly crave but everyone tells you is 'bad'. | Simple carbohydrates are useful, easy fuel. Complex carbs are slower but stable fuel and dietary fibre is good for the gut. |
| **Protein** | Steak and shakes … gym-junkie stuff. | Made of amino acids, which are essential building blocks of most things. |
| **Metabolism** | How quickly you process food. | All the chemical changes in your body that give you energy to function. |
| **Water** | World's most boring drink that everyone tells us we don't have enough of. | Another nutrient that you desperately need and don't have enough of. |
| **Alcohol** | World's best drinks. | Empty calories, as in they give you energy that can be burned or stored but also lack nutritional value. |
| **Breakfast** | The most important meal of the day, right? | Whatever meal is the first meal of the day that 'breaks' your 'fast'. |
| **Health** | You need this more than anything else. | You need this more than anything else. |

# Dr Krista and her eureka moments

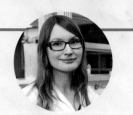

We know IF works for weight loss because of our own life experience, and because so many of our readers/members have achieved such incredible results, but we also know because of clever people like Dr Krista.

Krista is actually a professor of nutrition at the University of Illinois, Chicago, and we profess that she's awesome. She's spent her entire career doing IF research and is the author of the *Every-Other-Day Diet*, which is alternate-day fasting and similar to our 3-day method.

When she started her research, there were only two human studies and a dozen animal studies. All the human studies were done on lean people so we guess you could say the scientific literature was slim pickings. (Someone get Vicki away from the keyboard.)

Seriously though, during her PhD and post-doctorate studies, Krista noticed that people really struggled with daily calorie restriction. Mostly because of all the food logging, they'd get burned out after about a month or two.

She started to wonder whether people actually had to diet every day to lose weight and whether restricting calories every other day would work. Her theory was that maybe this approach could propel them through a diet because they would get frequent breaks.

Krista's theory was proved right: people stuck to the alternate-day method. They liked it, and it worked!

Since then, Dr Krista has been involved in extensive further research to explore some of the health benefits of IF and we've been lucky enough to consult with her as we developed SFD.

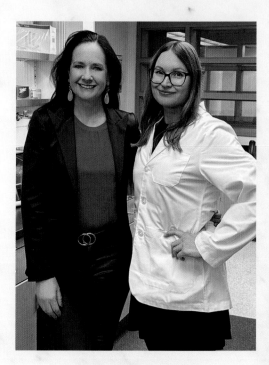

Victoria with Dr Krista in her laboratory at the University of Illinois, Chicago.

However, it's her brand-new findings that have brought us to this book, and she shares them with us all here, dispelling some fasting fables in the process!

*Read on to learn more about Dr Krista's top 5 eureka moments* ⟶

# Eureka moment #1

## (THE BEST ONE): YOU CAN LOSE WEIGHT AND REALLY ENJOY YOURSELF!

We've recently completed the world's longest-ever study into time-restricted eating: our study lasted for 12 months!

### THE OBJECTIVE:

To see if time-restricted eating (TRE) is better for weight loss and weight-loss maintenance versus daily calorie restriction (CR).

### THE EXPERIMENT:

Participants with obesity were randomly assigned to a group that would follow a traditional, calorie-restriction method of dieting; a part-day style of dieting (time-restricted eating); and a control group that didn't change their diet at all. For simplicity, let's call the groups 'traditional', 'part-time' and 'control'.

The **traditional group** reduced their intake by 500 calories each day and they could eat at any time. The **part-time group** could consume any food or drink between 12 pm and 8 pm without counting calories, but could only have water the rest of the time. (This is called 'water fasting'.) Of course, we encouraged eating a healthy diet, but for the study, no food restrictions or calorie restrictions were placed on the part-time group during the eating window.

The **control group** didn't change their diet at all, so that we can be sure that any weight loss seen in other groups didn't occur under 'normal' or 'control' conditions. The year of research was divided into six months of weight loss (the first half) and six months of maintenance. It's also the first study to examine the effect of time-restricted eating on weight-loss maintenance.

### THE RESULTS:

Weight loss in both dieting groups was between 5 and 23 kg but the most interesting and exciting finding is that those who did IF really enjoyed the whole process! They lost weight AND they reported that they would definitely be continuing this way of life.

In contrast, the majority who were on traditional every-day-low-calorie dieting couldn't wait for the 12 months to end and stated they would definitely NOT be continuing, even though they had lost weight. It was too hard and too sad!

Some participants asked if they could switch methods during the study (unfortunately not permitted), and many said they would be switching to the part-day method at the end of the study.

**Eureka! In short, this research indicated that IF using time-restricted eating is not only effective for weight loss, but it is also sustainable (and likeable) in the long term.**

## Restrictive vs. part-time

- There's very little point in following a restrictive diet if it is not enjoyable long-term because when most people 'go off the diet' they are highly likely to put the weight back on again.
- Part-time dieting on the other hand enables people to enjoy the foods and drinks they love, encouraging adherence and making it a sustainable lifestyle.

# Eureka moment #2

## YOU CAN LOSE WEIGHT EVEN WITHOUT COUNTING CALORIES

In the 12-month study, participants in the part-time group were not asked to count calories or restrict their eating in any way other than eating within an eight-hour window. The part-time fasters lost the same amount of weight as those that were eating 500 calories fewer than normal every day. But they didn't have to count calories at all, ever.

Part-time eating – that is eating within a window of six to eight hours – has been shown to really work for people because they stick to it! Weight loss is likely the product of a confined eating window that naturally cuts out calories and results in unintentional calorie restriction.

It's just such a relief for people to not have to constantly watch what they're eating and still lose weight.

**Eureka! If you hate the idea of counting calories or don't want to obsess over it, you don't have to and you can still lose weight.**

*It's just such a relief for people to not have to constantly watch what they're eating and still lose weight.*

## Counting calories

Although you don't have to count calories on our SFD program, for best results we DO recommend you keep count, especially in the beginning. This is because your portion sizes may be too large and sometimes the food and drink you're consuming may be WAY more calories than you ever imagined – it's actually quite shocking to many members when they start! After a while you get to know off the top of your head how many calories are in most foods and drinks so you don't have to be so diligent about counting. It becomes automatic.

# Eureka moment #3

## IF IMPROVES INSULIN SENSITIVITY AND TYPE 2 DIABETES CAN BE REVERSED

**THE OBJECTIVE:**

To see if time-restricted eating is a better diet than traditional calorie restriction to treat type 2 diabetes.

**THE EXPERIMENT:**

We randomly assigned participants with type 2 diabetes to one of three groups. One group followed a traditional calorie-restriction diet that reduced their daily intake by 500 calories. The second group followed a part-day style of dieting (time-restricted eating) that allowed them to eat anything between 12 noon and 8 pm but only water was allowed outside of that window. The final control group didn't change their diet at all. This study went on for six months.

The study isn't published yet, but our interim findings are hugely promising! So far, we are seeing that time-restricted eating produces twice the weight loss (5 per cent) versus traditional calorie restriction (2.5 per cent). It may also help to lower their HbA1c number (see below). The participants also say that an eating window is a refreshing alternative to constant calorie restriction and it is much easier to stick to. Many participants could come off some diabetes medication.

**Eureka! Better blood sugar! No matter what your weight, that's something everyone should be aiming for: insulin sensitivity that is as high as possible.**

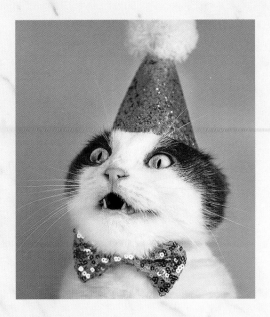

## Why insulin sensitivity is important

When you eat food and there's a lot of sugar in it, it goes into your stomach and eventually ends up in your bloodstream about an hour later. This is 'blood sugar' and too much sugar floating around your blood is really bad because it sticks to your red blood cells. It's what we refer to as glycated haemoglobin (measured as HbA1c) – a major diabetes risk factor. The higher the HbA1c number, the more glucose there is in your blood. Too much glucose floating around in your blood all the time without getting cleared away will wreak havoc on the body. You want to be sensitive to insulin because that is the signal for our bodies to take glucose out of the blood and put it to use as quickly as possible. Type 2 diabetes is when your body can't produce enough insulin or isn't sensitive to insulin.

## Eureka moment #4

### POLYCYSTIC OVARIAN SYNDROME (PCOS)

#### THE OBJECTIVE

The goal of this study was to see if eating within a daily time-restricted window could be used as an alternative to traditional calorie-restriction dieting to treat PCOS. Weight loss is the only proven method to improve hormonal profile and reverse PCOS.

#### THE EXPERIMENT

In this pilot study, we randomly assigned pre-menopausal women to one of three groups. There was a time-restricted eating group and a traditional diet group (both with the same regimens as our other studies) and a control group with no dietary changes. The participants were required to maintain their method for three months.

We found that eating within a window produced more weight loss and belly-fat loss than daily calorie restriction after three months in women with PCOS.

It also produced greater decreases in testosterone and free androgen index (an indicator of PCOS severity) compared to the calorie restriction group. Insulin sensitivity (remember, that's a good thing) also increased more in the eating-window group.

**Eureka! These findings suggest that an eating window may be a better diet to treat PCOS than traditional dieting. A large-scale study is still needed to confirm these findings and we're kicking one off now!**

## Treating PCOS

PCOS occurs when a woman's body releases too much testosterone, resulting in irregular periods, fertility issues and acne. Finding ways to treat PCOS is super significant for many women who suffer from it, so these results are encouraging.

# Eureka moment #5:

## TREATING FATTY LIVER DISEASE

Having fatty liver disease greatly increases one's risk of developing type 2 diabetes, but a combination of alternate-day fasting and exercise may reduce that risk.

### THE OBJECTIVE:

The goal of this study was to see if alternate-day fasting combined with exercise could help treat fatty liver disease.

### THE EXPERIMENT:

We randomly assigned participants with obesity and fatty liver disease to one of four groups for this three-month study. The first group did alternate-day fasting alone by consuming 600 calories on fasting days, which alternated with a day of normal eating in between. The second group was the exercise group, which had to complete 60 minutes of aerobic exercise (jogging or cycling) for five days a week. The third group did alternate-day fasting *and* the exercise regimen, while the final control group changed nothing.

### RESULTS:

We found that the group that combined alternate- day fasting with exercise significantly decreased liver fat by 6 per cent and improved liver enzyme profile over the three months. They also lost 5 per cent body fat while maintaining muscle mass. In addition, insulin sensitivity increased, which suggests that the risk of developing diabetes was lowered.

**Eureka! These findings show that combining exercise with IF is not just great for treating fatty liver disease; it also shows that fasting doesn't mean muscle loss.**

# The true and false of IF fables

We challenged Dr Krista to do some myth busting for us and you heard it here first. Diet fairytales? Exposed!

## FABLE #1

### REDUCING CALORIE INTAKE WILL PUT MY BODY INTO STARVATION MODE

This won't happen unless you're strictly fasting for several days. Your body needs energy for everything – even the most seemingly benign things, like sleeping and thinking. The number of calories your body needs to account for your physical needs, digestion and 'just be' depends on your weight and muscle mass, but as a general average that could be 1800. The fascinating thing is that 1300 of those calories would go towards powering those constant 'just be' processes.

So what happens when the body runs out of fresh calories to use?

If you reduce your caloric (and therefore energy) intake, your body will use whatever it can to keep those functions going. If you're not getting enough from your food because you're on a fast, it will use stored energy in your muscles or liver and eventually tap into the energy stored in fat. It won't save it for later, because it needs to function.

If you are eating a healthy diet while IF, your body will not go into starvation mode.

## FABLE #2

### WEIGHT LOSS WILL SLOW YOUR METABOLISM DOWN

This is true when you lose weight by any means. Your metabolism will technically decrease because your weight is part of what determines your metabolism. Remember, 'metabolism' is the amount of energy that your body needs to work – it's not how fast you process food. Your daily calorie needs will decrease as your body gets smaller so your metabolism does decrease, but this doesn't mean your body will slow the rate that it burns calories. It's also just as true to say that when you put on weight, your metabolism will increase, because it takes more energy to move more weight around, and if you eat more food at a larger weight, it will take more energy to process that food.

Genetic factors mean some people have a naturally higher metabolism than others – for example, some fidgety people will burn extra calories unconsciously (this is called non-exercise activity thermogenesis). Also, some people's bodies are more sensitive to an influx of food energy, so their bodies burn more fat at night.

If you're not counting calories and you have hit a plateau, it might be time to make sure you are consuming the right number of calories. If you think that your metabolism has decreased because your weight loss is slowing, check your TDEE again (see page 59). Your calorie needs may be much smaller than when you started because you've lost weight!

## FABLE #3

### INTERMITTENT FASTING WILL MAKE YOU LOSE MUSCLE

This is true ... but it's also true for any method of weight loss.

When a person loses weight, about 75 per cent of the weight lost is from fat and 25 per cent of the weight lost is from muscle. Any dietary changes that lead to weight loss will result in the same.

If you want to maintain muscle mass, make sure you're consuming enough protein and keep up your regular exercise such as weight bearing or lifting weights to keep building muscle up.

*There isn't any evidence that skipping breakfast is bad for your health!*

## FABLE #4

### SKIPPING BREAKFAST IS BAD

A review of scientific studies that examined the effect of breakfast on weight actually showed that people who eat breakfast weighed more than those that don't. This is likely because people that ate breakfast consumed 250 more calories per day, which makes sense because if you eat three meals a day, you eat more calories.

There isn't any evidence that skipping breakfast is bad for your health. Some studies suggest that the body is better at processing food earlier in the day so, if your lifestyle allows, you can shift your eating window so that it is earlier. But if doing that means you won't stick to your fasting window because it's too hard – don't do it.

There's nothing special about breakfast that makes it a 'must-have' meal for health, especially if you are overweight. Losing weight (even if it means skipping breakfast) is good for you.

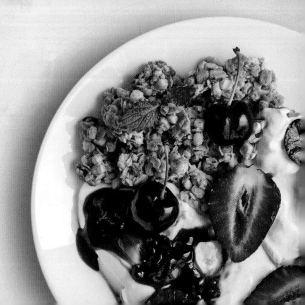

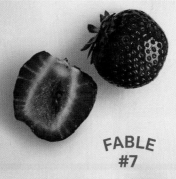

## FABLE #5

### I'LL HAVE NO ENERGY WHEN I FAST

Many people find the first 10 days of fasting hard, so don't be surprised if you feel a bit more lethargic than usual.

After that, most people actually feel energised during a fast and can even exercise in a fasted state.

## FABLE #6

### FASTING WILL KEEP ME UP AT NIGHT BECAUSE I'LL BE HUNGRY

In our review of studies that tested the effects of fasting on sleep, we found that it didn't affect sleep duration or quality. Although we didn't see any positive effects on sleep, we also didn't observe any negative effects.

## FABLE #7

### I CAN'T FAST BECAUSE I CAN'T LIVE WITHOUT COFFEE

What 'breaks' the fast is still fairly contentious among researchers, but for weight loss, having coffee during your fasting hours is fine.

We allowed the people in our research to consume coffee during a fast (with up to 1 teaspoon sugar and 1 teaspoon cream) and they still lost weight and experienced the same health benefits.

Be mindful that the extras you add to your coffee can increase calories, but ultimately if coffee is part of your life, you should find a way to work it in. The most important thing is that you can maintain your diet long-term, and if having a coffee outside of your fast helps, then it's not a bad thing.

Coffee drinkers rejoice! In the next chapter we show you exactly how to enjoy your 'part-of-life' coffee in the 'Clean fasts vs dirty fasts' section on page 57!

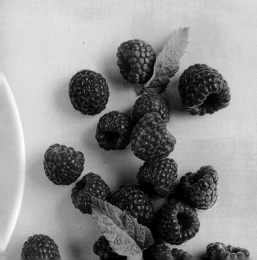

# Lessons from Dr Jason Fung

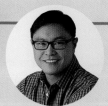

What about the real world? Does fasting work when you're not in a constrained lab environment and the call of fast-food drive-throughs rings out at almost every corner? *Spoiler alert* – it does. We asked another world-leading fasting expert, Dr Jason Fung, a practising nephrologist and author of *The Obesity Code* and *The Complete Guide to Fasting*, to take us through important IF lessons from his practice.

## LESSON #1

### THERE'S MORE TO WEIGHT THAN EATING

Telling someone what to do isn't enough. It's like saying, 'You shouldn't eat cookies!' That's good advice, but it doesn't mean I'm not going to eat the cookies, right? There are lots of reasons why people eat: it could be food addiction, emotional reasons, social reasons or they could eat because they're triggered by watching The Food Network.

You have to look at the underlying reasons behind what you're doing. This is especially important for weight-loss plateaus. If you're at a plateau, you have to change something and it isn't always a matter of changing how or what you eat.

## LESSON #2

### FASTING IS NORMAL

Fasting is simply a period of time when you're not eating and you're using energy that you have stored. It's natural. The very word 'breakfast' means the meal that 'breaks' your 'fast'. In other words, you have to fast in order to break your fast. It's just part of a natural cycle, like sleeping and waking.

If you look back at the 70s, most people were fasting for about 12–14 hours a day. You ate dinner (say at 6 pm) and maybe you ate breakfast at 8 am the next day. That's a natural cycle – a 14-hour fast that everybody did without even thinking about it. You have to balance the feeding and the fasting so it's not all feeding, and it's not all fasting.

## LESSON #3

### EATING CONSTANTLY HINDERS WEIGHT LOSS

It's impossible to eat and lose weight. Insulin inhibits lipolysis (fat-burning) and, when you eat, insulin goes up. If you're spending more time eating than fasting, you're spending more time storing calories than burning calories. That's just the way it is. If you're eating all the time, then you're giving yourself less opportunity to use that stored body fat as energy.

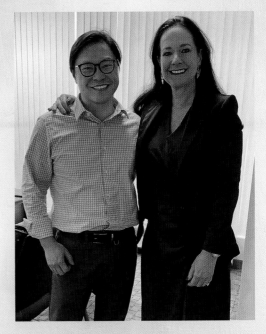

Dr Jason Fung is a Toronto-based nephrologist and world-leading expert in intermittent fasting.

## LESSON #4

### YOU WON'T STARVE

People think a lot about what they'll get deprived of when they fast. Fasting will deprive you of calories for some time, but if you have excess body fat, then your body has excess energy. If you think you'll be deprived of nutrients, eat nutritionally dense foods when you're not fasting or take a multivitamin. But from a medical standpoint, there isn't anything worrisome about fasting if you have weight to lose.

## LESSON #5

### FASTING DOES IMPROVE HEALTH

I focus mostly on treating people with type 2 diabetes because they are the people at highest risk of disease. We've seen incredible results. Sometimes people come in, and they've been on high doses of insulin for 20 years. We start them on the proper diet and fasting, and they basically come off everything and become non-diabetic. It's just a stunning reversal of their disease process, all within an extremely short period of time, which is incredible. We've seen the risk of heart disease go down, the risk of cancer go down, the risk of stroke go down – with fasting we were able to reverse that.

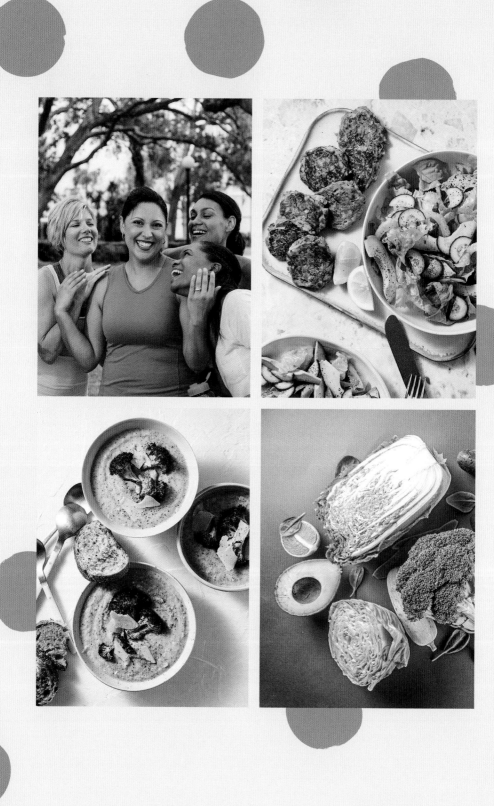

CHAPTER

3

# Supercharging your start

# The fastest diet – the first four weeks

Welcome to the start of The Fastest Diet – your supercharged start, in fact!

We've created a roadmap for your first four weeks, building up to the SFD supercharging method – the most powerful way to fast for weight loss without sacrificing your social life. We'll start by taking you through the 3-day (4:3) and 2-day (5:2) methods before adding in the part-day (16:8) method, so you'll get a chance to try your hand at all three and find the one that best suits you before you ... sound the trumpets ... supercharge!

Here's the plan:

| Week 1 – 3-day (4:3) method |
| Week 2 – 2-day (5:2) method |
| Week 3 – Part-day (16:8) method |
| Week 4 – Supercharge! |

By the end of the first four weeks, you can decide whether you want to stick with supercharging or ease off into one of the other methods. So flexy, baby. Get ready to do a happy dance when you find that, yes, you can so do this, and yes, you are seeing immediate results!

## Week 1

### THE 3-DAY (4:3) METHOD

In an ideal 3-day (4:3) method world, the best approach is to intersperse your fasting days with feasting days in between. Over a week, this could work with Monday, Wednesday and Friday being fast days and Tuesday and Thursday being normal days. This also leaves the weekend totally diet-free! Other people prefer to do three quick days in succession, e.g. Monday, Tuesday, Wednesday, then have four days diet-free. It's totally up to you how you want to mash this up.

**HERE'S HOW TO MAKE IT WORK FOR YOU**

On your fast days, consume half of your TDEE calorie allocation and on the off days you can eat your recommended TDEE allocation. Learn how to calculate your TDEE on page 59, or go to https://superfastdiet.com/what-is-tdee/. For most people, that works out to be 1000 calories, 3 days a week for women (1200 for men) and 2000 calories on the other 4 days (2400 for men).

This is the method that we recommend most people start with if they're unsure of which one to pick, as so many of our readers/members say it's the easiest one to do when you're unused to fasting. You can fit quite a lot into 1000 calories when you know how! As such, we think it's a great way to kick-start your four weeks but feel free to choose 2-day or part-day if you prefer.

# The 3-day (4:3) method in action

## Emma

**LOST** 27 kg    Size 18 to size 10

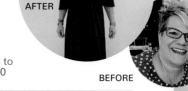

AFTER

BEFORE

Before she started SFD, Emma says she felt like a spectator in her own life. She constantly started new diets only to fail and feel more frustrated and depressed than ever. The 3-day method was a game-changer as it fit into her lifestyle 'rather than the other way around'. Now 27 kg later, Emma says she's gained her life back.

'When I was overweight, my mind felt it was in the wrong body,' Emma says. 'I felt like a spectator, always standing on the sidelines. I would spend my weekends tired and not having the energy to be fully immersed in my own family, hiding myself away under jackets and cardigans. I would start a new diet on a Monday, all guns blazing, but would then derail by the end of the week. After about two weeks, I would give up again. I was in this perpetual dieting hamster wheel!'

Emma decided to give SFD a try, although she was sceptical at first. 'I thought "This can't be the magic spell that I have been searching for" but after my first week I had already managed to drop 1.5 kg so I thought, "Wow! Maybe it is!" I think SFD is different because it not only provides you with an amazing way of eating but it is sustainable and can fit into your lifestyle instead of the other way around – probably why I had failed at everything else I had tried. I quickly could see SFD becoming my way of life and I didn't feel like I was "going without".

'I am a huge fan of the 3-day method because it brings a much needed balance into my life – I am really good for three days a week and enjoy my fasting days but I still have 1000 calories so I never feel deprived. Then on my non-fast days I can enjoy my wine and still have all the amazing foods I love; nothing is off limits and I find it easy to plan my calories if I am eating out at a restaurant, which I do once a week. I've dropped four dress sizes and I love clothes shopping now – no longer back of the rack, I used to hate that. I also now love my walking/exercise and do a minimum of five times a week. Unheard of when I started this journey. I have fallen in love with myself again and I feel confident – not the fake confidence when you put on a front but a real "show up and be present" confidence. I've gained my life back.'

**'I am really good for three days a week and enjoy my fasting days ... Then on my non-fast days I can enjoy my wine and still have all the amazing foods I love ... I never feel deprived.'**

# Week 2

## THE 2-DAY (5:2) METHOD

In an ideal 2-day (5:2) method world, once again the best approach is to intersperse your fasting days with feasting days in between. Over a week, this could work with Monday and Wednesday being fast days and the rest being non-fasting days. Other people prefer to do a quick two days in succession, e.g. Monday, Tuesday, then have five days diet-free. Once again – totally your call.

### HERE'S HOW TO MAKE IT WORK FOR YOU

On your fast days, consume one-quarter of your TDEE calorie allocation and on the off days you can eat your recommended TDEE allocation. Learn how to calculate your TDEE on page 59 or go to https://superfastdiet.com/what-is-tdee/

For most people, that works out to be 500 calories, two days a week for women (600 for men) and 2000 calories on the other five days (2400 for men).

### NOTE

Even if your TDEE says to go below 500 calories on your fast day we recommend eating the full 500 as it's too hard otherwise and it will still work for you.

### HERE'S OUR ABSOLUTE SUPER-HOT TIP

Plan, plan, plan. The easiest way to tackle your first 2-day fast day is to have all your food planned ahead. The less time you spend in the kitchen the better, lest the fridge and pantry start whispering your name. (Surely it's not just us ...?)

Having your meals ready to go means that you don't have to think about your food – or worse, try and shop on a fast day. Ugh. You can also divvy up your calorie allowance between meals and snacks prior and spread them out so it feels like you're eating more.

With the average example for a female of 500 calories, you might spread them out like so:

| |
|---|
| **Breakfast:** 50 calories (probably a small coffee or tea) |
| **Mid-morning snack:** 60 calories |
| **Lunch:** 150 calories |
| **Afternoon snack:** 40 calories |
| **Dinner:** 200 calories |

If you think that delicious meals that are low-cal are impossible, flick to the recipes at the back of this book and get ready to salivate.

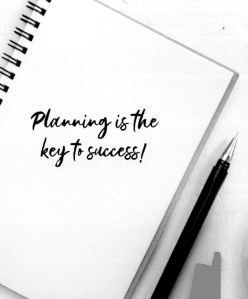

*Planning is the key to success!*

# The 2-day method in action

## Chris

  LOST 15.5 kg    Size 18 to size 10

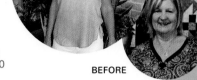

AFTER

BEFORE

Prior to trying the 2-day method, Chris constantly felt uncomfortable, usually dressing in big jeans and baggy tops. She says she was definitely ready for a change, so when her sister saw a TV ad for SuperFastDiet and called saying, 'I think I've found something that will work for you', Chris decided to give it a try. After losing 15.5 kg, she describes the decision as 'life-changing'.

'My sister had seen me struggle for a long time and I was very unhappy with my weight,' Chris says. 'I'd tried just about everything but nothing worked. All that changed when my sister rang. I started the 2-day method the very next day.'

'I got immediate results,' Chris reports. 'I enjoyed controlling and restricting calories on the fasting days and not feeling deprived, then being able to eat normally on the other five days. I feel empowered, in charge of what I'm doing. It feels amazing to be off that rollercoaster of weight coming off and going back on again.

'I love the lifestyle as it is so simple to fit into my everyday life. I actually look forward to my fast days because two days a week is really easy to prepare for. You just have simple meals for the day, like a big pot of vegetable soup that I boil up in winter, or big salads for lunch and dinner in summer, then I have some protein for sustenance, like eggs or chicken. I'm not hungry, and I know the next day I can have whatever I want.'

Chris has lost 15.5 kg, two dress sizes and approximately 30 cm in measurements. She says her skin has improved too and she now feels comfortable and happy with herself. 'It's life-changing. I love what I see in the mirror and I'm confident for the first time in a long time. Everyone around me notices how much happier and content I am. It's the best feeling ever.'

**'I actually look forward to my fast days because two days a week is really easy to prepare for ... I'm not hungry, and I know the next day I can have whatever I want.'**

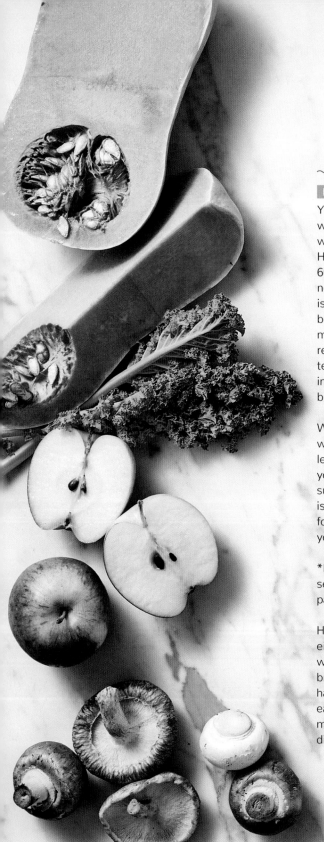

# Week 3

## PART-DAY (16:8) METHOD

**PART-DAY IS VERY STRAIGHTFORWARD**

You eat all of your food within an eight-hour window on all days. Your eight-hour eating window can be placed anywhere in the day. However, research suggests that waiting 60 minutes after waking before you eat and not eating for 2–3 hours before you go to bed is beneficial (but not crucial). This is partly because our bodies generally have increased melatonin levels at those times. Melatonin reduces insulin release (the hormone that tells your body to process food), so without insulin, your body isn't great at digesting big meals.

When you're in your eight-hour eating window, you should consume 20 per cent less than your TDEE (learn how to calculate your TDEE on page 59 or go to https://superfastdiet.com/what-is-tdee/), which is about 1600 calories for women, 2000 for men. When you're out of your window, you should only consume water.*

*Don't panic ... (we see you, coffee drinkers) see the Clean fasts vs dirty fasts section on page 57!

Here's how to make it work for you. Pick an eight-hour eating window that suits your life, whatever time of day that may be. If you love breakfast, that might be 9 am–5 pm and you have an early dinner. If you can skip breakfast easily, that might look like 1 pm –9 pm (the most popular choice as it enables you to eat dinner with the family).

# The part-day
# method in action

## Nicola

**LOST** 13 kg

Size 14
to size 8

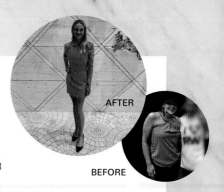

AFTER

BEFORE

Nicola felt she was just going through the motions in life. Battling health issues then gaining weight had left her with low self-confidence and, no matter what she tried, nothing worked. Then she discovered the part-day method and 13 kg later, she describes herself as finally 'free'.

'Before SFD I felt that I had lost my sparkle,' Nicola says. 'I was going through the everyday motions, but I had lost some of my mojo, especially after my illness. On the outside I hid how I was feeling by wearing bright-coloured lipsticks, accessories and baggy tops but my self-confidence was low.'

When asked about what other diets she's tried, Nicola says, 'What haven't I tried? But I would always lose weight then put it all back on again, plus some.'

Enter SFD and the part-day method! 'The difference about SFD was that I felt like I wasn't on a "diet". I could eat what I wanted, have a social life and still lose weight. It was too good to be true!

'The part-day method suits my lifestyle. I've never been a huge breakfast lover, so it wasn't a big adjustment for me. Also, I like to socialise and have nice dinners with family and friends, and I exercise most days, so I need more calories throughout the day, which the part-day method allows for.'

Nicola says she has regained her self-confidence and is excited to dress up each day. 'I can go to my wardrobe and put anything on! I no longer have that small section in my wardrobe where only a few clothes fit. I'm happy, confident, and free from the shackles of a "diet mentality". It's a feeling of freedom. It's very liberating.'

Nicola has noticed improvements in her wellbeing as well. 'Apart from the weight, I have noticed a significant improvement in my health markers. As a breast cancer survivor, I have regular blood work done. My cholesterol and blood pressure are all in the healthy range and my visceral fat (the fat around my organs) has improved significantly. I feel enthusiastic about life again!'

**'The part-day method suits my lifestyle. I've never been a huge breakfast lover, so it wasn't a big adjustment for me. Also, I like to solcialise and have nice dinners with family and friends.'**

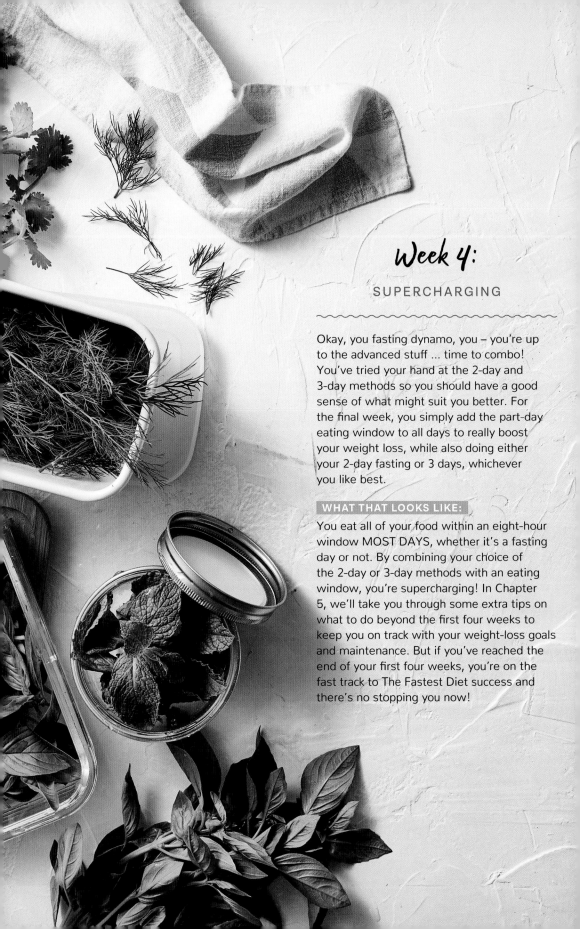

## Week 4:

### SUPERCHARGING

Okay, you fasting dynamo, you – you're up to the advanced stuff ... time to combo! You've tried your hand at the 2-day and 3-day methods so you should have a good sense of what might suit you better. For the final week, you simply add the part-day eating window to all days to really boost your weight loss, while also doing either your 2-day fasting or 3 days, whichever you like best.

**WHAT THAT LOOKS LIKE:**

You eat all of your food within an eight-hour window MOST DAYS, whether it's a fasting day or not. By combining your choice of the 2-day or 3-day methods with an eating window, you're supercharging! In Chapter 5, we'll take you through some extra tips on what to do beyond the first four weeks to keep you on track with your weight-loss goals and maintenance. But if you've reached the end of your first four weeks, you're on the fast track to The Fastest Diet success and there's no stopping you now!

# Supercharging in action

**LOST** 31 kg

Size 18
to size 8–10

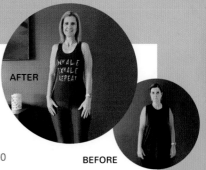
AFTER

BEFORE

Fiona had got to 'that stage' with her weight. Embarrassed and feeling desperate, Fiona was considering gastric sleeve surgery but decided to give SuperFastDiet a try. Now, after losing a staggering 31 kg, she has a whole new outlook on life. She credits 'supercharging' with accelerating her results.

At a size 18 and weighing over 93 kg, weight gain was destroying Fiona's life. 'I was embarrassed about my weight and had got to that stage. I would avoid getting my photo taken and hide up the back – I didn't really even look at myself in the mirror.'

Fiona decided that SuperFastDiet was her last chance to give it everything she could without surgery and she quickly realised that IF was the game-changer she'd been searching for. 'I had only ever been on diets that lowered your calories but having the fasting days and non-fasting made it so much easier to stick to long-term. I found the 3-day method really worked for me – 1000 calories is so much food once you get a few favourite low-cal meals into the routine. Preparation is key – my friends call me the "Queen of Prep"!

'I then heard about supercharging results by combining methods so I delayed eating breakfast and ate within an eight-hour window on my three fasting days, essentially making them 3-day and part-day fasts. The weight fell off even quicker and it was so easy, I now eat within an eight-hour window most days to maintain my results.'

Fiona is now down to a size 8–10 and sustains it with ease. She's also found other benefits to her health and lifestyle that she never expected.

'I am not getting back pain anymore, my menopausal night sweats have stopped and my fitness has improved. I am living with happiness and self-acceptance now. It's given me my life back.'

**'I heard about supercharging results by combining methods so I delayed eating breakfast and ate within an eight-hour window on my three fasting days, essentially making them 3-day and part-day fasts. The weight fell off even quicker.'**

# 'Dirty' fasting in action

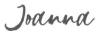 *Joanna*

**LOST** 35 kg

 Size 18 to size 10

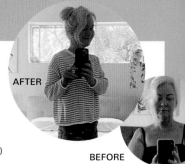

AFTER

BEFORE

Prior to starting SFD, Joanna describes herself as 'sad and out of alignment'. She had no energy and shied away from social situations, yet nothing seemed to work when she tried to lose the weight that was literally weighing her down. Then she discovered part-day fasting ... but with a twist. Now 35 kg later she calls it her 'dirty little secret'.

'I felt lifeless before SFD,' Joanna admits. 'I tended to wear cardigans to cover my arms and woke up exhausted every morning, forcing myself to push through. I was playing small in life.

'I tried shakes and deficit eating among many other things but SFD was so different. I immediately got results in the first two weeks, then six weeks in I slept through the night for the first time in years. That was it for me. I knew it was my forever lifestyle.'

Joanna attributes it all to the part-day method ... plus a dirty little secret. 'It's so adaptable and versatile, and cost effective as you don't need any special foods or supplements. Then there's the dirty fasting bonus. I love, love, love being a dirty faster! Basically, it means you can cheat by having 50 calories of whatever food and drinks you like during your 16-hour fasting window, which might not sound like much, but it can be!

'I have lemon water, long blacks, bowls of vegie broth and ½ cup blueberries or strawberries, all while still not technically breaking or slowing down the effectiveness of my fast. My clients who I now coach in IF enjoy milk in their tea, an almond latte, broth, berries, jelly, cucumbers, corn thins with a slice of tomato ... as long as it's under 50 calories they can go for their life!'

Asked how she feels now, Joanna says everything has changed. 'I have an energy and a zest for life again. I could be blindfolded and put my hand in my wardrobe and everything fits. I now live life fully, every day.'

**'I love, love, love being a dirty faster! Basically, it means you can cheat by having 50 calories of whatever food and drinks you like during your 16-hour fasting window, which might not sound like much, but it can be!'**

## Clean fasts vs dirty fasts

Should you keep it clean or do it dirty? In other words, do you have to be 'perfect' outside your eating window or can you be a bit naughty?

**KEEPING IT CLEAN =** Having only water, unflavoured sparkling water, herbal tea, black tea, black coffee or bone broth outside your window. We say they're 'clean' because they're all sort of clear. Some like to take it a step further and consume only water – if you can do that, we applaud you! In fact, if you fast 'clean' at all, well done – but don't worry if that sounds too hard as most of our members like it 'dirty'!

**LIKING IT DIRTY** If you think you'd rather something less transparent than those clean options, then 'dirty' fasts are for you. During a dirty fast, you can consume up to 50 calories outside of your window and yes, our experience shows you will get away with your naughty little secret, i.e. you'll still lose just as much weight! The 50 calories could be a drink such as a small almond milk cappuccino, tea with a splash of milk, a cup of broth or miso soup or sparkling water with a hint of flavour. It could be food, too – a handful of strawberries, carrot and celery sticks, lite jelly. We've had thousands of SuperFasters do the part-day method and dirty fast with great results. This is one of those crutches that can help you when you get started, or for days when you just can't. Because, you ... can.

## Ready? Set? Goals!

Okay, this is the SUPER exciting bit – envisaging your new life! Setting goals is mega important because if you don't know what you want ... how can you stay motivated to get there?

### DECIDING YOUR WEIGHT-LOSS GOAL

In general, a weight-loss goal that is between 5 and 10 per cent of your current body weight is recommended to start with. That is also an initial range of weight loss that has proved realistic and feasible with IF in scientific studies.

Once you have achieved your initial goal you can set another, then another. Nothing motivates like success and Gen found this really worked for her when she started on her path to losing a large amount of weight: 'At first, I just set myself the goal of losing 5 kg as trying to achieve a 35 kg weight loss just seemed too daunting. Breaking it down into smaller goals seemed a lot easier and it was. I lost the first amount easily then I decided to lose 5 kg more. Then I did it again, and again. Seven times, in fact. At every milestone I celebrated and rewarded myself in some way, which made the whole experience incredibly positive. I liken it to climbing a mountain and pausing at intervals to enjoy the view. It makes all the difference to pat yourself on the back and realise just what you are actually achieving along the way. It kept me focused and encouraged and by the time I stood on the pinnacle of my weight-loss journey I truly appreciated just what I'd done, and I was proud of myself for each and every step of the way.'

Setting milestones like this is incredibly important psychologically and a great way to do this is by using what's known as the '**Six C Cycle**' (see over the page).

# Six C Cycle

**1 Capture** This is where you capture your ultimate goal in your mind, imagining how it will feel to get there, what you will wear, where you will go and who will be with you. This is your BIG goal and your ultimate dream.

**2 Chunk** This is where you chop it up into actionable, realistic and measurable little goals starting with the first realistic, 'not-too-huge so yes, I can do that' achievement e.g. 5 kg.

**3 Clear** Get negative thoughts/naysayers/ old habits out of the way! This is where you clearly identify any actions you need to take to get you to your goal. Write them down each day if that helps e.g. Greek salad for lunch and get away from the fridge at 6 pm by going for a walk.

**4 Commit** This is where you set a timing goal – not a scary one, an exciting one! For example: 'By the end of the month, I will have done three weeks of IF and will be writing down my new measurements and weight.'

**5 Complete** This is when you go out and achieve that first milestone!

**6 Celebrate** This is when you revel in your success and reward yourself. HOORAY!

This is what your Six C Cycle might look like in the first four weeks:

**1 Capture**
Dream big.

**2 Chunk**
Plan for your first milestone of the four weeks, four methods.

**3 Clear**
Get those new habits firmly in place.

**4 Commit**
It's only four weeks – get focused on the outcome!

**5 Complete**
Fasting, feasting and living your IF life!

**6 Celebrate**
Wow – look what four weeks can do! I'm off for a facial!

And so you begin your next Six C Cycle and focus on your next milestone towards your BIG goal.

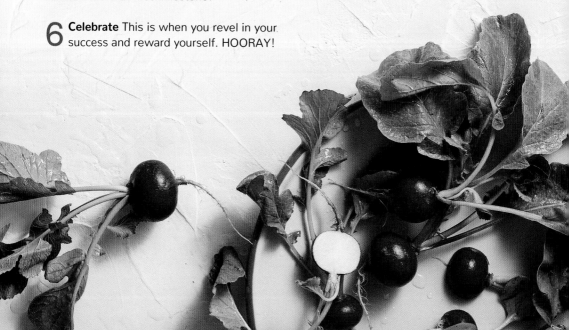

# Your starting point

With your goals and your Six C Cycle in place, now it's time to measure. The first thing we're going to do is calculate that calorie estimate for your body we keep talking about, your Total Daily Energy Expenditure (TDEE).

Now you don't have to do this; however, your TDEE will give you a much closer indication of how many calories you need to function day-to-day than the usual general estimates – e.g. a 1000-calorie fast day might come out as 974 calories for you. #superpersonalised

TDEE takes your gender, weight, height, body-fat percentage and activity levels into account. We use the TDEE equation called the 'Mifflin-St. Jeor Equation'. It was developed in 1990 and has been validated by various studies as well as nutrition professionals as the most accurate way of estimating caloric needs. The American Dietetic Association thinks that it can accurately measure resting energy expenditure to within 10 per cent. Pretty clever, huh?

## TDEE FORMULA FOR FEMALES

### Step 1

Calculate BMR (basal metabolic rate) using the formula below:
BMR = (height in centimetres x 6.25) + (weight in kilograms x 9.99) – (age x 4.92) – 161

### Step 2

Calculate TDEE (total daily energy expenditure)
TDEE = BMR x activity level

**Sedentary** (little to no exercise) BMR x 1.1

**Lightly active** (light exercise/sports 1–3 days/week) BMR x 1.275

**Moderately active** (moderate exercise/ sports 3–5 days/week) BMR x 1.35

**Very active** (hard exercise/sports 6–7 days a week) BMR x 1.525

## TDEE FORMULA FOR MALES

### Step 1

Calculate BMR (basal metabolic rate) using the formula below:
BMR = (height in centimetres x 6.25) + (weight in kilograms x 9.99) – (age x 4.92) + 5

### Step 2

Calculate TDEE (total daily energy expenditure)
TDEE = BMR x activity level

**Sedentary** (little to no exercise) BMR x 1.2

**Lightly active** (light exercise/sports 1–3 days/week) BMR x 1.375

**Moderately active** (moderate exercise/ sports 3–5 days/week) BMR x 1.55

**Very active** (hard exercise/sports 6–7 days a week) BMR x 1.725

**Extremely active** (very heavy exercise/ physical job/training twice a day) BMR x 1.9

Many people overestimate their activity levels. For optimum weight-loss results, you should select your minimum weekly activity level, rather than your maximum or average. And, if in doubt, choose 'sedentary'. (Sorry, but it's true. Our modern lives often fall short of their 'active' design potential. We can't all be Ms Trog running away from lions and chasing mammoths.)

**Maths not your thing? Save your brainpower and head online to use our free TDEE calculator. Go to https://superfastdiet.com/what-is-tdee/**

**IS THIS RIGHT? MY TDEE ALLOWS FOR WAAAY LESS THAN 500 ON A 2-DAY FAST DAY**

If you're petite or not very active, your calorie allowance for a 2-day fast day could be under 500. If this is the case, we recommend using the general guide of 500 calories. You'll still lose weight!

*You are much more than a bunch of numbers or a photo!*

## Love yourself enough to measure up

If scales, mirrors, measuring tape and before photos freak you out, you're not alone. We've had the 'scale scaries' too. But to get to where you're going, you need to know where you're starting from, so these steps are important.

It helps to remember this: you are much more than a bunch of numbers or a photo. We bet there are so many things to love about you. Are you insanely creative? Do you choose super thoughtful gifts? Do you give 100 per cent to your kids? Do you have the best sense of humour? All those things are you, too. Write them down before you look in the mirror or step onto the scales. Then, if you feel a negative thought creeping in, remind yourself of all that you are, and that you're making a huge, positive change here to feel even better about the amazing person that makes up you.

Love yourself enough to measure, weigh and click away with your camera. Just think how good it's going to feel when you do this again in four weeks' time! Besides, it's just for you. It's not like this is going to be your new Facebook profile pic or anything. (Something Gen may or may not have accidentally done when she wasn't wearing her glasses.)

**BONUS TIP:**

Weigh yourself first thing in the morning, naked, before coffee/tea. Sans wet hair. Maybe take off your earrings too ... mmm and before you moisturise even! Ha-ha, Vic says 😌

# Tracking your progress

Yes, the main focus is actually achieving that four-week, four-method challenge, but seeing your progress is the fun stuff! Think back to that mountain: you are here to climb it but taking photos and knowing how far you've come is the actual experience. It's not only about the destination, it's also about the journey, and there's so much to enjoy as you travel along.

There are lots of ways to do this and here are a few things to consider:

**1 It isn't only about you, scales.** Sometimes scales aren't the best indicator of your progress. Translate that to you – if you feel and look slimmer than before, but step on the scales and see that the numbers haven't changed, this could be because you've started exercising and put on 'heavy but healthy' muscle. Take that, scales! It could also be that you are holding extra fluid for some reason or other, or it could be hormonal. Either way, don't let those scales get you down!

**2 The camera does/doesn't lie.** You only have to look at some of the before/after photos of our case studies in this book to see how motivating snapshots can be, but the camera won't tell the whole truth unless you make sure you're comparing apples to apples. Try wearing similar clothes in a similar place at similar angles to get the most accurate shots of your progress. Even this can be subjective, however, so it's important to motivate yourself with the truest possible measurement: er, measurement.

## HOW TO TAKE YOUR MEASUREMENTS

**BUST:** around bra-strap level, directly across widest part of bust/chest

**ARM:** 10 cm above elbow

**NATURAL WAIST:** across smallest part of waist, around 2 cm above belly button

**WAIST:** line up top of measuring tape with bottom of belly button

**HIPS:** across widest part of the hip (generally where hip and bottom meet)

**THIGH:** 15 cm above knee

How you keep tabs is totally up to you. We've created the perfect, personalised weight-loss portal inside our program where you can record absolutely everything. Alternatively, a spreadsheet or diary will do the job, but there are also some handy apps that can help you along, as listed below.

- **Activity trackers.** An Apple Watch, smartphone, Fitbit, pedometer app or Strava can be great for tracking your daily activities and understanding your habits.
- **YouTube.** Sometimes you just need to see baby animal videos you know? We've also created some IF content and popped it on there, too – youtube.com/superfastdiet
- **Calorie counters.** Apps are helpful databases that can do all the calculating for you. You can also go low-tech and use an actual calculator/notebook or your phone to track your calories. Or you can just go off our meal plans and make it super easy. We'll go over calories and how to not count calories in later chapters so don't stress. You'll have options.

## Your tribe

Like anything big in life, having your closest people supporting you is super important. And what could be more important than your health and happiness? Make sure you avoid negative nellies, especially ones who'll consciously or unconsciously try to sabotage you. ('What are you doing that for?', 'Here we go again' etc.) and tell your loved ones (especially those living with you) why and what you're doing so they can encourage you to make these amazing changes in your life. It also helps if you get them onside with any menu tweaks that you put in place, too.

Speaking of which, here's some good news: you won't have to make a separate meal for yourself and your family. In most cases, you can prepare (or have someone else prepare) a large meal and amend your portion to suit your calorie allowance, letting the other members of the household go nuts! If you're using the recipes in the back, they really will because they're totally delicious! You can also swap out traditionally heavy sides to make your family faves more fasting-friendly.

Here are some fasting with family food swaps that we love:

### BONUS TIPS FOR STAYING OUT OF THE FAMILY-FOOD TRAP:

- Pack your own snacks (nuts are a great option), to keep you from munching on processed sugar-loaded snacks.
- Try to break the habit of finishing your kids' food.
- If the rest of your household is demanding snacks (it happens), buy things that you don't like to make it less tempting for yourself. Or better yet, take them out for a single-serve treat (and feel free to have one yourself too, if you wish) so that you don't have to bring any tempting treats into the house.
- It also helps to have the support of people who are in it with you. And thanks to the internet you can connect with thousands of them by joining SuperFastDiet at www.superfastdiet.com

| Family fave | Fasting friendly |
| --- | --- |
| Traditional fettuccine (approx 350 calories per 100 g) | Konjac pasta (approx 35 calories per 100 g) |
| Traditional flour pizza base (approx 300 calories) | Part flour, part cauliflower pizza base (approx 70 calories) |
| White rice (approx 130 calories per 100 g) | Cauliflower rice (approx 18 calories per 100 g) |
| White burger bun (approx 173 calories) | Ditch the bread and wrap your burger in a crunchy lettuce leaf (1 large lettuce leaf is approx 2 calories) |
| Crispy taco shells (approx 65 calories per shell) | Hey, come on! At only 65 cals each Taco Tuesdays are a fasting winner! |

## How to fly through your very first fast day

You can't hurry love, or a fast day, but there are a few things you can do to make it feel like it's flying by. We've helped tens of thousands of people and collected tonnes of tips for how to make it through your very first fast day without overthinking it/obsessing over food.

Here's some of our best:

- Be like Gen and tell yourself you can eat whatever you like the next day to make it through.
- Plan for non-food related activities like spending the day in the park, at the beach or window shopping (far, far away from the food court).
- Distract, distract, distract! Afternoon slump making you crave sugar? Go for a walk instead of reaching for the cookie jar.
- Drink plenty of water, including sparkling, which is even more filling. We recommend aiming for 2.5 litres a day. Carry your drink bottle with you.
- Find and collect motivational mantras/funny quotes and post them in key places e.g. the fridge door.
- Treat yourself to a manicure or pedicure.
- Play with your kids or pets.
- Get an early night. It's great for getting more sleep and waking up to a new day of normal eating sooner.

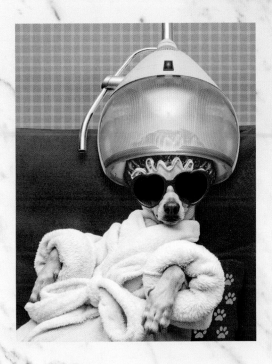

*Getting a manicure & pedicure? Great – treat yo' self!*

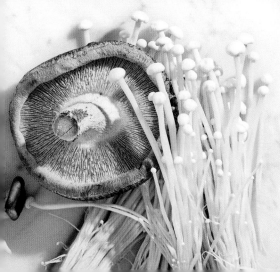

Since rejoining in September 22 I have lost 8.5 kg and am very happy with my progress. I love the SFD community as it is so encouraging, helpful and friendly and there is always someone to help. I have changed so much; I have strength and I believe in myself. I am going to finish my journey. I want to thank SFD family, the coaches I have had and of course Gen and Vic for their fantastic program. I just love this way of life.

**HELEN REIDY**

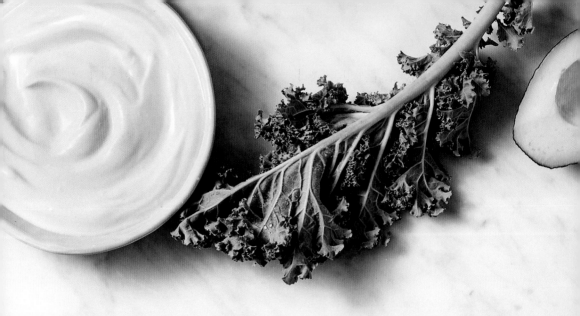

## FOOD TIPS FOR YOUR FIRST FAST DAY

- Meal prep like crazy. You can even label everything and portion it all out in advance if you're a bit OTT or really into your Tupperware collection.
- Also, cook the day before so that you can spend as little time in the kitchen as possible. If you're an ingredient snacker, you'll get why.
- Write out your menu for the day with timing spread out so that you can clearly see when food is coming. Or just have your big bag of food at the ready in the fridge. Again, dependant on whether you're OTT or NOTT.
- Choose super yummy foods! The recipes in the back are all de-lish, so you really can't go wrong. When you start on a health kick, it can be tempting to do all the healthy things, all at once. For example, you might want to pick the healthiest-looking recipes and cook up a storm. We're all for that, but it might be easier to choose a recipe that is close to (at least in flavour and cuisine) meals that you're used to. For example, if you don't usually eat salads, choose a low-calorie stir-fry or roast instead.
- Pack snacks. A little snack can go a long way between meals. Broth, berries, apples, boiled eggs and soups are some of our faves.

## WHAT NOT TO DO

The modern world has more food traps than Indiana trying to find his way to the temple. You'll get better at resisting temptation as you get used to fasting, but in the beginning:

- Don't try and scroll time away on social media if you're into food porn.
- Don't watch the clock. That's fasting torture. If you're doing the part-day or supercharging method and (rightly) want to know when your window is open, set an alarm.
- Don't go grocery shopping when you're hungry. Just. Don't.
- Don't be too hard on yourself if you don't make it through. Change is rarely easy and how your body responds or adapts to fasting will be different to others. If your first day ends with a #fastfail e.g. an accidental wine/takeout fest with hubby, that's totally okay. We've had lots of people go through a whoops! on their first day and press on with great success the next time they tried. Give yourself permission to try and fail, then try again. #noguilt #nojudgementhere

#startagaintomorrow

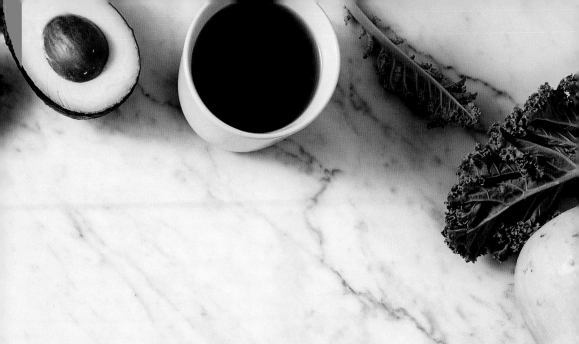

# Troubleshooting your first four weeks

### WHAT TO DO IF YOU KINDA #FASTFAIL BIG TIME?

If your first four weeks didn't exactly go to plan, that's okay too. Life happens. The important thing to remember is that you have given this your first shot and you can now give it another. Because guess what? There's no deadline here. You have goals, you have dreams, you have great plans and an awesome solution at your fingertips, yes, but there's also a person living a whole life and you are allowed to be human.

We've had some of members/readers who've hit an early roadblock such as a work crisis/personal crisis/um-I-went-on-a-spontaneous-holiday and pretty much failed at their first attempt, sure. However, nearly all of them went back and had another shot and are now LOVING this way of life.

The point of the first four weeks isn't perfection; it's to sample what methods work for you and what doesn't. So yep, just hit your reset button and let's try that again.

### DO I NEED TO TRY BOTH 2-DAY AND 3-DAY?

Ideally yes, you should try all the methods so that you can see what suits you best.

### CAN I JUMP RIGHT INTO SUPERCHARGING?

Absolutely yes! If you're feeling bold and want to dive straight into the supercharging method – go for it! This is probably the method that will take the most getting used to because you're applying an eating window and some fast days. But don't let that put you off! If you think you can keep the supercharging method up long-term, go ahead. But don't be afraid to adjust things along the way if you feel like another method would suit you better. And definitely don't give up on IF altogether if you find that supercharging wasn't for you. It's just one option and any of the methods are going to give your fast and fabulous results, regardless. We have countless success stories from those who have only done one method the whole time and they just love that particular method! Give them all a go if you can and see what works best for your lifestyle.

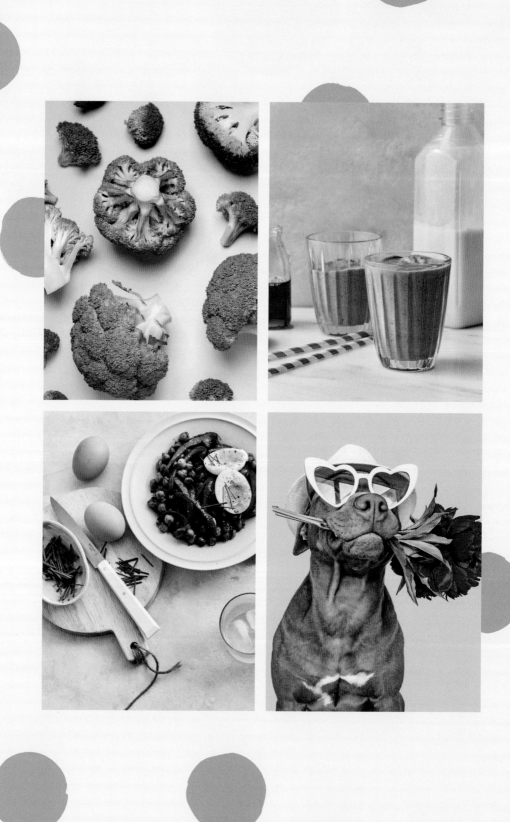

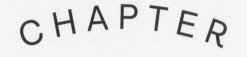

CHAPTER

4

# Food, glorious food!

# Food, what is it good for?

Food, ha, get down, what is it good for?
Absolutely everything! Say it again.

If you haven't caught onto the fact yet ...
we love food!

Food is satisfying and nutritious, comforting
and delicious. It's crunchy, it's creamy, it's
sweet and it's steamy. It's tangy and sour,
and with spice it has power! It's literally the
salt-of-the-earth stuff of life and we savour
every mouthful.

It's little wonder we get a bit obsessed with
cooking shows. Combine that with travel
scenery and you'll find us glued to the TV,
spellbound by the exotic flavours of the
world and all the spiritual, cultural and social
aspects that come with one of the greatest
pleasures in life: eating.

We love to eat out, taste new foods or just
sit back and watch *The Great British Bake Off*,
which is why we love intermittent fasting (IF)
– because you don't have to give up all the
foods and drinks you enjoy on a delay/indulge
way of life.

This entire chapter is dedicated to this
wondrous fact as we explore every aspect
of the essential, sensory act of eating – one
of the most enjoyable aspects of our DNA.

## Eating is for nutrition, health, taste and fun!

But more specifically, it's how we get energy
and nutrients. Now, nutrition may not always
be on your mind when you sit down to eat
something scrummy, say ... oh we don't
know ... how about a banana and chocolate
sundae? Some part of your health-conscious
mind might immediately start justifying your
choice with thought-mail such as:

*'It's got ice-cream. That's calcium, right
there. And a banana. They're packed full
of fibre and potassium, not to mention the
nuts that are good for you too, right? And
chocolate is really just cocoa which comes
from a plant – which makes that essentially
salad ... so what if there's ten tonnes of
sugar and fat in here? It's practically a health
shake. Yes, it's a protein sundae with a side
salad. They should sell these in gyms.'*

Ah yes, food justification. If they gave out
awards for this practice, we'd both need to
have trophy rooms built in our houses. Gen
has a BFF who calls her on this, cutting her
off with comments like: 'Oh, come on. It's
a zillion calories. Just enjoy it.'

And BFF makes a very good point. Hey, if
you're not fasting and it's somewhere within
your calorie estimate for the non-fasting day,
do just enjoy it.

But it also brings us to that word: calories.
It's enough to strike fear into the heart of
many a serial dieter but in truth, it's actually
just another tool.

## Jim

 **LOST** 24 kg

 Size 44 to size 36

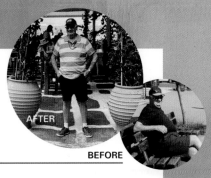

AFTER

BEFORE

Jim Young began his fasting journey with the encouragement of his wife, Sue, who had already begun dropping kilos on the SuperFastDiet. Sue's health was dramatically improving with intermittent fasting, with both her blood pressure and cholesterol down. As Jim was suffering from kidney problems, his doctor recommended he lose weight as well. 'I saw how much weight my wife was losing and once the doctor said I needed to lose weight, I just copied what she was doing.'

Jim eased himself into the part-day method over a couple of weeks, extending his fast time so he could start at 12 noon and finish by 8 pm: 'I never felt hungry and weight actually came off from the first week. I went on to lose 10 kg in the first three months and the doc was very impressed.'

Jim says his tips are to 'keep busy and always have healthy good choices available', and to 'stop buying potato chips and eating fried foods'. He has enjoyed multiple benefits from this way of life: 'I have more energy and I still enjoy all the foods I like. I feel good about myself too – going from a size 44 trousers down to a size 36, and I've also cut many centimetres off the leather on my belts.'

His doctors continued to be amazed by Jim's progress. 'The diet was working so well that, at one time, my GP was worried about how much weight I was losing. He asked me: 'Are you sure you're just doing what Sue is doing and deliberately losing weight? It's not because you are sick?' He tested me and my health was great! My kidney specialist keeps wanting to talk about how I did it, as he needs to lose weight himself.'

Jim likes that he has inspired those around him to lose weight and improve their health as well: 'My daughter is now taking in her clothes as she's lost weight inspired by Sue and me, too.'

It's little wonder Jim has motivated others. He began his weight loss journey at 110 kg and now weighs 86 kg. As he says, 'If I can do it in my late seventies, with no real idea about food or nutrition and no exercise other than daily movement, anyone can. The simplicity of this plan makes it something I can do for the rest of my life.'

**'I never felt hungry and weight actually came off from the first week … the doc was very impressed.'**

Your body needs calories to power itself up for such things as thinking, breathing, moving, digesting. However, calories aren't the be-all and end-all of food choices. On top of getting energy from food, your body also gets nutrients from food. These are the chemicals that it needs to build tissues, repair things and send signals between organs and body parts so that it can function. Also important.

There are also two types of nutrients that your body needs: micronutrients and macronutrients.

Micronutrients are only needed in teeny-tiny amounts (hence micro). These are things like vitamins and minerals. Macronutrients are needed in larger amounts (hence macro). These are proteins, fats, carbohydrates and water.

Knowing how much to give your body can be tricky, and that's okay. Don't feel pressured to have it all figured out before you start The Fastest Diet. We're going to show you just how easy-peasy it can be to make every-bite-count by making good choices when it comes to calories and nutrition, helping you to lose weight and still enjoy that great love of your life: food. #havingitall

## Kilojoules or calories?

The amount of energy we get from food is measured in calories. Sometimes you'll see energy measured in kilojoules (kJ) instead (if you can read such things on those tiny food nutritional labels). For simplicity's sake, we speak in calories, but if you ever do manage to read the label and have to convert kilojoules to calories, you can roughly just divide by four.

## JERF

If you take just one nutritional bit of advice from us, this is it: JERF it.

**JERF = Just. Eat. Real. Food.** That is, fresh food rather than processed. Not all the time of course because, you know, cake, but try to make it a general rule of thumb whenever you can. Taking a prehistoric leaf out of the book of Ms Trog just makes sense, biologically. It's what we're built for, and if it didn't come straight from nature, well then where did it come from?

Some factory that's chucked in a whole other bunch of stuff to make you want to eat more, that's where. Processed foods are manufactured products – it's in the maker's best interest to make you want to keep eating. One study compared the effect of processed food to unprocessed food that proved the point. The researchers made sure the meals were matched for calorie content and the same amount of protein, carbohydrates, fat and fibre. Even so, at the end of the study (which was tightly controlled in a lab), they found that the people who were fed processed food ate about 500 calories more than the unprocessed group, and they put on weight. Wow, right?

Weight loss aside, we need to eat more real foods for good health. In 2022, the Australian Bureau of Statistics reported that less than half of Australian adults were meeting their recommended daily serves of two or more pieces of fruit. Only 8.7 per cent met the recommendation of five to six servings of vegetables each day. Fruits and vegies are fantastic sources of nourishing nutrients, are generally free from preservatives and chemicals, and often contain fewer calories than processed foods.

Plus they can be filling. And they are totally yummy. One thing we found when we started IF and needed low-cal foods on fast days was that fruit and veg were our best option, allowance and nutrition-wise. Lo and behold, we fell in love with the fresh, crunchy taste of food grown and picked straight from the earth and watered by the rain. It's almost like you can taste the sunshine! We got so adept at being creative with salads and vegie dishes we now eat them purely for pleasure on non-fast days too. You'll see what we mean in the recipe section. #youdomakefriendswithsalad #flowerpeople

**HEALTH FACT**

Fruits and vegetables are loaded with phytochemicals that can reduce inflammation, assist detoxification and may even reduce cancer risk.

Different vegetables come with different beneficial nutrients, so to help your body get all it needs, go for variety. This could be as simple as keeping a base of leafy greens in your salad (rich in folate that's essential for healthy cell growth and function) and adding two different vegetables each time you plate up. This will help introduce a variety of nutrients into your system and give your taste buds a range of wonderfully different experiences, especially when you play around with fresh herbs, fruits and condiments. Yum!

## ALL THE PRETTY COLOURS ...

Another simple solution to having a more JERF diet is to eat the rainbow! The availability of certain phytochemicals in a fruit or vegetable is thought to be influenced by its colour, so eating a rainbow of fresh foods will help add variety to the nutrients that you eat. Besides, what would you rather eat? Boring, bland mush on a plate or food bursting with colourful life? #somewhereovertherainbow=health

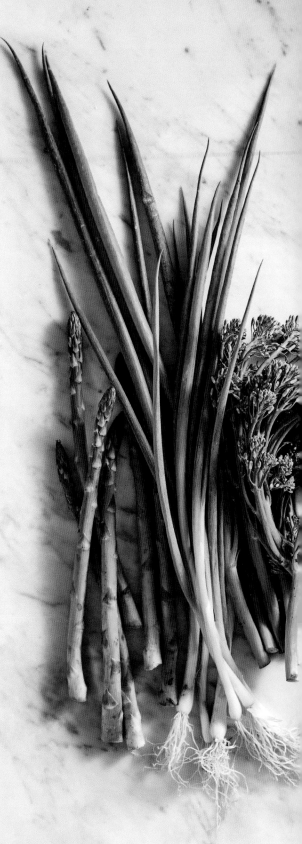

# Rosemary

**LOST** 14 kg  Size 14 to size 8

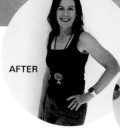

AFTER

BEFORE

Socialiser Rosemary found herself withdrawing from outings and activities when she gained weight, feeling so down she hid herself away. Discovering SFD changed everything, and she lost 14 kg while rejoining her social life. She's now living life to the fullest.

'Before I joined the SFD family, I was generally very unhappy with my weight, the way I looked and particularly how I felt,' Rosemary says. 'Whenever I was going out somewhere, I struggled to find the right clothes. I felt so down on myself. I withdrew and removed myself from all the social outings and activities that I would normally be involved in. I had low self-esteem. I was depressed and generally very unhappy. I have tried all sorts of different diets and also thought I knew what I should and shouldn't eat – problem was I didn't stick at anything and lost heart quite quickly. I would drop some weight and then put it all back on again.' Then along came SFD: 'I got results from week one.'

Rosemary soon started socialising again and the weight kept falling off. 'I love that it gives me the freedom and flexibility to still enjoy being social – going out for dinner, attending various events and not having to go without the food and drinks I love. I was still able to go away on wine and dine weekends and not feel guilty.

'Having discipline on my fast days and flexibility on my non-fast days makes SFD perfect for a socialiser like me. I love the 3-day method as it is easily manageable, and I love my weekends being out and about. I never felt that I was going without. Mon–Thurs were non-alcohol days and then on weekends I could still enjoy my glasses of champagne. When I started to become more active and involved again socially with my friends, there were so many compliments. I still get heaps now and it's been over 12 months.

'I feel fabulous and so happy within myself. I also carry myself differently and know that this has an impact on how people interact with me. At 58 years old, I am the healthiest I have been since I was in my late thirties. I am mentally and physically ready to take on what the next 20 years has to bring. I'm living my life to the fullest!

**'I love the 3-day method as it is easily manageable, and I love my weekends being out and about.** I never felt like I was going without.'

# Eating for fullness vs overeating

Not many people think to pause during a meal and ask themselves, 'Are we there yet? Are we there yet? Are we there yet?' like they're a kid on an eating journey, excited about reaching fullness-town. We're usually far too busy enjoying the experience of eating itself to really be aware of satiety, aka feeling full. No, fullness usually seems to hit us in an unexpected 'where did that possibly come from' way, and we're often surprised to find our tummy's suddenly protesting like Scotty in Star Trek. I canna give her any more, Captain.

'Why didn't you tell me?' we could well lament as we begin to moan and place a confused hand on the Magic Pudding-like bulge that's uncomfortably appeared in our middle. Oh, but your body did. It sent you very clear signals that you left hunger at the side of the road a long, long way back on this eating journey but you didn't seem to notice it had gone. You were too busy paying attention to that other, self-indulgent sensation: taste.

Here's what you missed while you were overdoing it at the flavour party with Mr Taste. In your mouth, his sensory cues of texture, flavour and bulk were keeping you distracted while your engine-room tummy stretched and became full/hydrated to capacity as it tried to cope with that motherload of nutrients. It told the brain-bridge on you but you weren't listening until it was too late and now you're left groaning in food-over regret.

This isn't just eating until you feel full; this is straight past the fullness sign into overeating land, yet it's very understandable stuff. We all do it – after all, Mr Taste is a very charming dinner companion. But there are some steps you can take to ensure this doesn't happen very often anymore.

1 **Slow down.** Pause and take a sip of water often, giving your body time to register the fullness signals. Some nutrients are only sensed in the gut, and it takes time for your food to get there. It's great advice to stop eating when you think you are 80 per cent full because it takes around 20 minutes for your brain to register your fullness.

2 **Chew.** If you break food down properly by chewing, it has a better chance of getting processed faster and sending those signals.

3 **Choose filling foods.** This may sound obvious but of course if you actually choose filling foods that are good for you, you'll eat less overall. You're still eating for taste, just smarter.

It's actually a good idea to eat for fullness, as long as it doesn't descend into overeating. Having enough protein is a great start, as protein makes you feel fuller for longer, reducing your food consumption later on. Eating enough fibre and good fats will help fill your stomach and JERFing in general is also a good idea because eating a variety of foods high in vitamins and minerals will satisfy your body's nutritional needs.

## EATING FOR FULLNESS ON A FAST DAY – YOUR POWER KEY TO SUCCESS

Filling foods are, of course, imperative on a fast day as you need everything you eat to fill you up as much as possible. Satiety really matters when you're talking a 500 or 1000 calorie allowance.

Satisfy any unhealthy cravings you might experience with healthy, low-calorie foods that contain a similar taste to what you crave; that way, you're more likely to feel satisfied and 'good' full. For example, if you're hankering for meatballs, try our Lemon Caper Chicken Meatballs (page 171), or if you want a cheesy dessert, give the Cucumber Cream Cheese Sandwiches (page 208) a go.

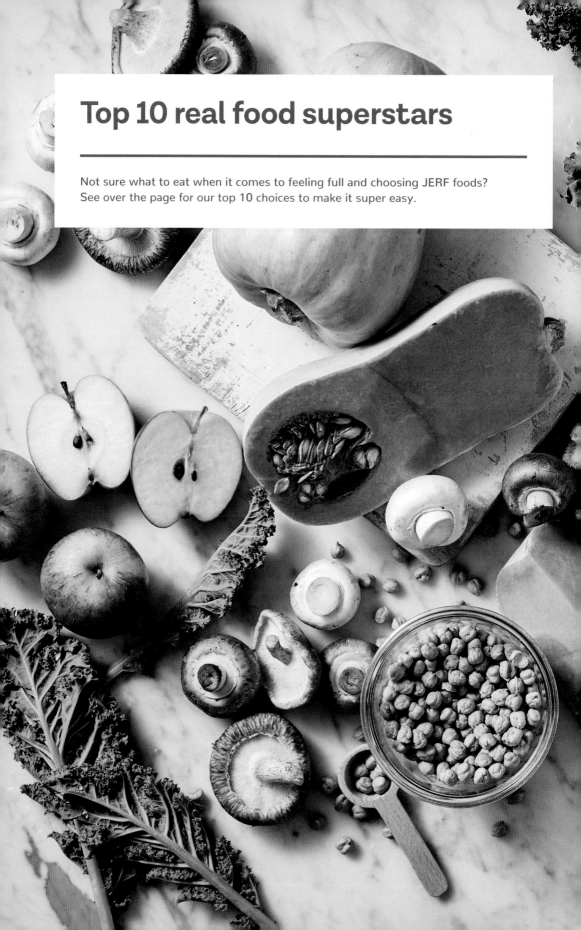

# Top 10 real food superstars

Not sure what to eat when it comes to feeling full and choosing JERF foods?
See over the page for our top 10 choices to make it super easy.

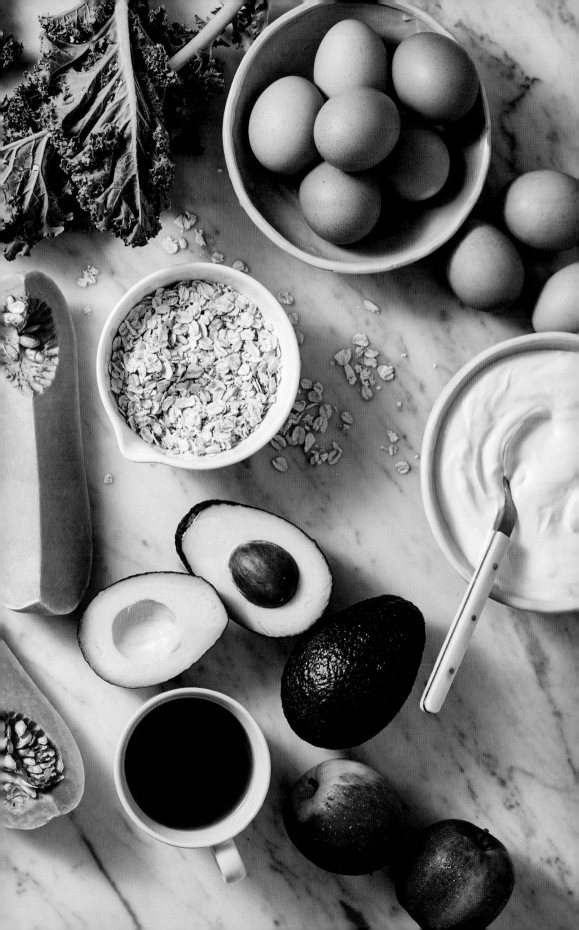

## Eggs

Eggs are a great satiating food because of their high protein content. They're also a great source of biotin (aka vitamin B7), which is important for the body to be able to break foods down into their nutritious little bits during digestion. Eggs are also a good source of vitamin A that supports white blood cell production and healthy bones. A medium boiled egg contains approximately 77 calories, making eggs a handy hunger-saving and low-calorie snack. Plus you can take them anywhere! – although we bags not sitting next to you on the bus.

## Avocados

Avocados are one of the best plant-based sources of healthy (monounsaturated) fats around and can improve blood cholesterol and ease inflammation. They also contain potassium (essential for cell hydration), magnesium (important for loads of chemical functions in the body) and folate (important for producing healthy red blood cells). Avocados are also rich in vitamins E, C and K, B vitamins and antioxidants. They are calorie-dense (approximately 300 per avocado), but if you add them to meals as slices, they make up for it with their nutritional magic.

## Yoghurt

Yoghurt has been a diet staple for yonks! It's rich in protein and calcium, which is vital for healthy bones, muscles and nerve functions. It's also rich in riboflavin, a B vitamin that's important for cell growth, and vitamin B12 that keeps your brain and nerve cells functioning. Yoghurt is versatile and can be added as a healthier alternative to cream in soups, dolloped on Mexican foods in place of sour cream, or served with fruits as a creamy dessert. Opt for non-flavoured, plain yoghurt like Greek yoghurt as there are generally fewer added calories. If you want to flavour your yoghurt, do so with fresh fruit instead. Or honey. Mmm mmm.

## Oats

Oats are an excellent source of fibres that are great for gut health and keep you feeling fuller for longer. One of these fibres is beta-glucan, which can also help clear cholesterol from your body. Oats contain phenolic compounds and phytoestrogens that can have an antioxidant effect on the body and reduce inflammation. Look for the least processed (like oat bran) as instant versions sometimes contain added sugar. #oats=goodbloat

## Kale

Once the superfood du jour and for good reason. Kale contains vitamins K, C and A, B vitamins, folate and fibre. It's a cruciferous vegetable, and others in this group (bok choy, broccoli, cauliflower, cabbage and brussels sprouts) are worthy of this list too. This is because they contain glucosinolates that get broken down into compounds that can reduce inflammation and protect healthy cells. Like most vegies, kale is low-cal at only 34 calories per cup. Try baking the leaves in the oven with a little sea salt. Totally delicious, trust us.

## Apples

A humble classic. Apples are a great source of fibre and vitamin C. They also contain quercetin, a chemical that has antioxidant and anti-inflammatory effects. Apples are also a good source of pectin, a fibre that helps with digestion and may also help lower 'bad' LDL cholesterol. An apple a day really does keep the doctor away when it comes to you know ... flushing your digestive system clean. Ahem. Just be sure you keep the skin on because that's where a lot of the goodness – and happy inner plumbing – comes from!

## Mushrooms

Historically, mushrooms have been used medicinally because of their healing properties. (Not that kind of medicinal use. Behave.) Now we know that mushrooms contain loads of healthy nutrients like B vitamins, potassium, selenium (good for DNA and healthy thyroid function), vitamin D (crucial for bone health) and phosphorus (helps regulate muscle and nerve function). Mr Mushroom is also very low in calories at only 15 calories per cup, leaving you so mush-room for more food in your cal allowance you'll be just loving this fun-gi on your fast days. (That's it Vicki. Go stand in the non-typing corner.)

## Butternut pumpkin

This underrated vegetable packs a nutritional punch as a source of vitamin C, vitamin B6, magnesium and potassium! Butternut pumpkins are versatile and can be incorporated into a bunch of dishes (like roasts, soups or frittatas). Texturally, they're not too far from potato (especially mashed) and are a great option for a high-protein and high-fibre side. Plus they are super, super low in calories at only 30 calories per cup! We often put roasted cubes over salads with a little crumbled feta, pine nuts and beetroot. So good.

## Tea

Yes, it's a drink, but tea is in our top 10 because it is rich in polyphenols – naturally occurring compounds that have antioxidant effects. Different teas contain different polyphenols: green tea contains epigallocatechin-3 gallate, black tea contains theaflavins, and herbal teas will have different polyphenols depending on the plant that they come from. All are believed to have health benefits. And, if taken without milk or sugar, a cuppa contains less than 2 calories – but if you need to add a splash of milk, go right ahead, you dirty faster, you!

## Chickpeas

A pulse that packs some nutritional punches! Chickpeas are an excellent source of starchy carbohydrates (pow!), protein (pow!) and B vitamins (pow!). They contain a soluble fibre called raffinose too, which can promote the production of the fatty-acid butyrate that can reduce inflammation in your guts. Chickpeas also contain amylose, a starch that is hard to digest and can help reduce spikes in blood sugar. High fibre and protein content make chickpeas another wonderfully satiating ingredient. With only about 119 calories per 100 g, they're a super nutritious, low-calorie way to add bulk to meals. We add them to all sorts of salads and dishes but they do work an absolute treat in a hot curry. Ka-pow!

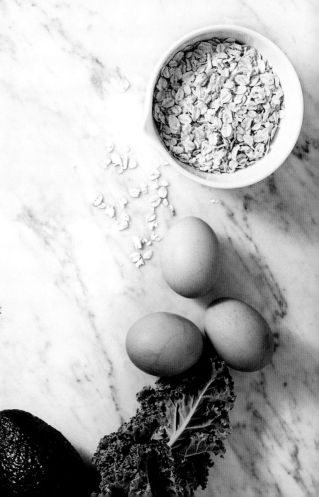

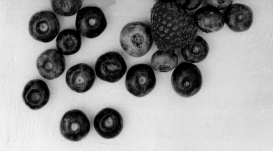

## How to outsmart the quicki-mart

Some people love grocery shopping, others hate it, but most have fallen into those impulse-purchase-at-the-counter, junk-food traps. We're not going to lie, we've left the shops with our fair share of half-price cheesy snacks and two-for-one bags of chockies, but we're a little more SFD-wiser these days. Here are a few of our BIG how-to outsmart the quicki-mart tips.

*Google the nutritional values ahead of time at home & not in the supermarket aisles!*

### Top tip #1
#### TROLLEY TACTICS

Never. Shop. Hungry. Ever, ever, ever. You know it won't end well if you let your rumbly tummy and Mr Taste forget past differences and get in cahoots behind that trolley.

On top of planning when to shop, you should also have a solid idea of what you're shopping for. Making a list based on your weekly meal plan will keep you on task at the shops and help eliminate the need to browse. We said 'help'. We know it's not easy getting past the junk-foods aisles, especially with Mr Taste/your tummy steering at the helm, but stay focused! A good rule to follow is: 'I'll get everything on my list first, then, if I could still be bothered to go back once I'm at the checkout, I will.' But you probably won't. Another rule of thumb is to try not to take the kids shopping with you, or naughty friends/partners who sneak things into the trolley when you're not looking. #temptationaborted

If your meal plan includes shopping for a packaged food you haven't used before, try googling the nutritional values ahead of time at home. It's a lot less awkward than being found scratching your head in the supermarket aisle by an old flame, squinting at those minuscule panels in blurry confusion.

### Top tip #2:
#### PERIMETER DWELLERS

All the JERF food – vegetables, fruit, dairy, meat, fish and health foods – are usually at the perimeter of the store, not in the aisles. And no, we don't know why this is. Some Trog family hunter/gatherer instinct still lurking in the supermarket management/ design team perhaps? It does seem to make sense that's where the best prey would roam, dwelling out there on the wild frontiers. As such, the bulk of your shopping time should be spent there but when you do need to venture into the shiny centre aisles of temptation, remember: Stick. To. Your. List.

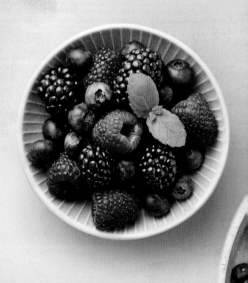

## Top Tip #3:

### USE THE RULE OF THIRDS

If you haven't had a chance to properly prep, an easy hack is to use the rule of thirds. Put simply, it means that if you glance at your shopping trolley, it should be balanced equally between:

⅓ **fresh vegetables and some fruits:** Leafy greens, beans, berries, starchy root vegetables, wholegrains, citrus fruits, stone fruits and cruciferous veggies like broccoli.

⅓ **meat, dairy and protein:** Eggs, yoghurt, milk, cheese, tofu, fish, lean meat and plant-based proteins.

⅓ **perishable:** Low-calorie/clever carb sides (e.g. konjac noodles, brown rice or quinoa), olive oils, condiments (sun-dried tomatoes and olives), bone broth and soups, coffee, tea and low-calorie crackers or popcorn.

Okay, this is a pretty perfect trolley, and oh, wouldn't it be great if that old flame should run into you preening at the checkout now, but let's get real: this is a part-time diet, and if there's a couple of treats in there too, that's fine! Life's too short for zero chocolate/ ice-cream. Let's just call it 3/3ds a perfect trolley + a treat or two. #SFDlife

## Counting calories ... or not

If the term 'calorie counting' sends a shiver down your spine, you're not alone. It's the hallmark of a lot of traditional diets and may have negative connotations if you've tried and failed at them before. We get it. It's not the be-all-and-end-all of fasting (especially if you're doing the part-time method on its own), but it is worth counting calories if you want to absolutely guarantee results, especially at first, and here's why.

There's no escaping the reality that your body needs calories, but too many will lead to weight gain. It's the old calories in/calories out rule, and while that simple equation is mostly true, there are easier ways to lose weight than sticking to this old dinosaur info alone.

Now here's where it gets a little sciencey but bear with us as we try to explain it in SFD-speak. The number of calories in foods represents how much **energy** your body can get, but that also depends on how your body **digests and absorbs** the energy from that food. This can vary depending on the amount of **fibre** consumed with food, how it's **cooked** and even a person's **gut microbiome**. (Little microbes running around in your gut that affect the whole process. Trust us, it's a thing.)

While knowing the calorie content of food is a great guide that we encourage to get the best results, it's not the be-all-and-end-all of what happens to food when you consume it. And it's definitely not the whole picture when it comes to weight loss – because it isn't just what you eat that matters, as you know by now, it's also when.

Having said all of that, we still think it's important to count calories, especially in the beginning, and make them **really** count. Let's put it this way: if you could only wear four items of clothing, maybe you would wear a dress (because it covers top and

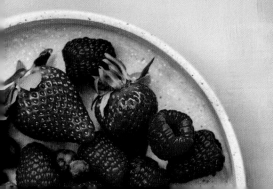

bottom), shoes, underwear(!) and a jacket for protection. You wouldn't waste your clothing allowance on handbags, heels and fancy earrings, even if they were your favourite pieces because, well, you'd be almost naked.

Your calorie allowance is much the same. You could pick your favourite foods on a fast day, e.g. a hamburger and fries, but you'd be pretty dang hungry for the rest of the day. (And they'd have to be a pretty small hamburger and fries if it's a 500-cal day.) One of the best things about SFD is how we've managed to resource and put together a huge range of low-cal foods and drinks that will give you soooo much more for your calorie buck ... and make that calorie allowance really count.

## IN THE BEGINNING

As we said, counting calories during your four-week start is recommended. It's the best way to ensure that you are keeping within your TDEE allowance, and the best way to get accurate about calorie values in foods. In our experience, 'guesstimating' makes it harder to get results.

Counting calories is also great for building a solid sense of what fits into your fast day and normal day calorie recommendations, i.e. discovering your go-to fast-faves. For example, you may come to realise that you really like pumpkin mash as an alternative to mash potato and it has a lot fewer calories, so that becomes a regular side.

You'll also get a sense of what foods are giving you energy, what foods are filling you up and what foods are/aren't worth the calorie tag. (Spoiler alert: JERF foods nearly always are worth it.)

As you get familiar with your new lifestyle, you can become more relaxed about calorie counting, knowing you can re-visit it anytime you need to, for example, if you hit a plateau and want to lose weight faster.

The point is that you don't know unless you know, you know? So yep, during your first four weeks, start by counting.

## CALORIE-COUNTING TOOLS

Technology is making counting calories pretty easy these days with some apps boasting the ability to count calories based on a picture of your food or the barcode of an item, and you can often search for the exact brand of food or ingredient you are eating. #clever

Measuring cups and spoons are ideal for measuring out the right portions (and recipe success). A kitchen scale is also great too.

## KEEPING IT IN PROPORTION

Once you've built up a good sense of the calories in your food, you can use more relaxed techniques to guide your portions. The 1, 2, 3, 4 approach uses your hand, a plate and four simple rules to help build a well-balanced meal. These are:

1 palmful of protein. Red meat servings should be about the size of your palm (without your fingers). Chicken, fish and tofu servings should be the size of your palm with fingers included.

2 handfuls of vegetables.

3 No more than $\frac{1}{3}$ of your plate should be filled with carbs.

4 Use a maximum of 4 teaspoons of fat, butter and oils.

An important caveat is that this rule only applies to servings of healthy, real foods like proteins, vegetables, nuts, fruits and complex carbs. The calorie count (and nutritional value) of refined food carbohydrates is incredibly varied so, again, it's best not to guesstimate. (Hey, it's a word in SFD world.)

## 1000-CALORIE SHORTCUT

Another one-to-four rough guide can be applied to the average 3-day fast day allowance of 1000 calories. That is:

100 calories for snacks

200 calories for breakfast

300 calories for lunch

400 calories for dinner

= 1000 calories for the day

## 100-calorie snacks

Snackaholics might feel slightly freaked out at the thought of a 100-calorie snack allocation. That's fair, considering a 100 g blueberry muffin is about 300+ calories(!). But if you're savvy about what snacks you choose ,you'd be surprised how much you can fit into a fast! Here are a few examples of small-serve and larger-serve values of lower-calorie snacks for each 'food-mood'.

*Be snack-savvy, you'd be surprised how much you can fit into a fast!*

| Mood | Okay | Really good |
|------|------|-------------|
| Chocolate-y | White chocolate (with more milk and less cocoa powder, white chocolate has less of the health benefits and more calories at approx 140 per serve) | 85 per cent dark chocolate (one serve approx 115 calories, so it's a bit over 100, but dark chocolate also contains heart-healthy flavanols so we'll let it slide!) |
| Crunchy | Salt and vinegar chips (approx 120 calories per 25 g serve) | Air-popped popcorn (approx 85 calories per 100 g serve) |
| Fruity | Dried mango (approx 100 calories per 30 g serve) | Mango fruit (approx 60 calories per 100 g) |
| Dippy | 1 tablespoon tzatziki dip (approx 18 calories) + 6 baked crackers (approx 102 calories per 20 g serve) | 1 tablespoon tzatziki dip (approx 18 calories) + ½ cup/60 g carrot sticks (approx 20 calories) |
| Fizzy | Lemonade (approx 109 calories per 250 ml serve) | Lemon-flavoured lightly sparkling water (approx 2 calories per 1.5 litres) |

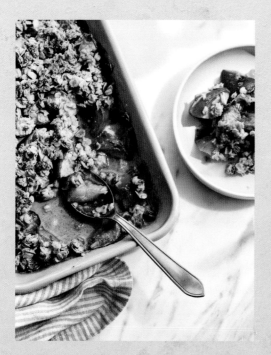

## Oh, sugar ... our sweet love affair

We know we can't have too much sugar because excess carbohydrates get stored as fat. And we also know that some sugars (the complex and starchy kind) are better than others. So how can we eat it and not throw our healthy-eating effort out the window?

A good start is to keep consumption below the World Health Organization's recommendation of 6 teaspoons of sugar per day or 24 grams. According to the latest ABS statistics, the highest consumers of sugar have at least 100 grams of sugar per day and make up 25 per cent of the population. This is equivalent to at least 23 teaspoons of naturally present or added sugars. Yikes! Too much sugar consumption can lead to insulin resistance, type 2 diabetes and weight gain.

It's everywhere, and often hiding in foods we wouldn't expect such as tomato sauce! In Australia, sucrose (a simple sugar extracted from sugar cane) is used widely as a sweetener, flavour enhancer and preservative for processed foods and drinks.

Our simple advice? When it comes to sugar, JERF it as much as possible. This includes eating fruit as nature intended – as a whole fruit, rather than dried or juiced. Why? Because when you process fruit by drying or juicing it, you're removing beneficial things like water or fibre and leaving mostly sugar.

While it's true that the sugar in fruit (fructose) is natural, to your body it is still a simple sugar and will elicit the same spiky response. The tricky thing about fructose is that our body sends it to the liver to be turned into fat, rather than using it as energy. This could be because in the age of Ms Trog, fruit was rare, so when we did stumble across it our bodies wanted to hang onto that energy bounty. These days, fructose is just one of the many sugars that we consume regularly, so it adds to an oversupply of energy. To peel

### WHAT IF I REALLY, REALLY DON'T WANT TO COUNT AT ALL ...

If you're really not into the idea of counting calories at all, ever, then we would recommend doing the part-day method.

Even though SFD recommends 20 per cent less calories within the eight-hour window, Dr Krista's study (see Chapter 2) showed her participants did lose weight anyway, even without counting calories. They also kept it off and reduced belly fat and blood sugar levels.

If you're going to choose this method without counting calories, we would really encourage aiming to consume a smart balance of macronutrients as best you can. You shouldn't expect to lose weight as quickly as you would by supercharging, but you will still lose weight.

SFD has done the work for you in the recipe section of this book regardless, which are all low in calories anyway – and are de-lic-ious.

this story back to basics? Eat fruit as a whole. And don't go too bananas.

A similar logic applies to wholegrain carbohydrates (brown rice, oats and wholegrain flour) and refined carbohydrates like white rice, white bread, cake and biscuits. Eating the wholegrain version means that you get some starch and fibre with the husk. Eating the refined version means you're eating a stripped-down sugar. And in a sweet baked dessert with toppings, you're adding sugar on sugar!

You don't have to cut refined sugars out altogether (how does one actually live without pavlova or carrot cake?), but do see them for what they are: not-that-healthy, calorie-laden albeit yummy special treats. So treat them as treats. Save them for special occasions and savour each bite. And day-to-day? Turn to fruits for a more nutritious source of sweetness.

By reducing the amount of sugar you have or opting for less calorie-dense alternatives (yep, artificial sweeteners – see the next section), you slowly change your palate and teach it not to expect the sweet stuff. Over time, your taste for what is sweet will change and you'll be wanting less sugar. #wekidyounot

### SUGAR ALTERNATIVES

Most discussions on artificial sweeteners involve wading into treacherous, debate-y waters. But we're going to do it because we think it has its place. First, let's remember that they are a very low-calorie alternative to traditional sugar. A teaspoon of sugar has 16 calories and a teaspoon of artificial sweetener like Splenda has 3 calories. Huge difference. Let's also remember that sugar is a taste that most people love. So, if we're trying to lose weight, are artificial sweeteners a useful tool or one we should avoid? It's a big question, so we asked Dr Krista.

'The scientific literature is a little messy on whether or not artificial sweeteners like those in diet soft drinks are good or bad for you. There is no concrete evidence that it spikes your insulin. A couple of studies show that it might, but most don't. What it does seem to do though, is increase sugar craving

'Limiting artificial sugars is a good idea if you want to minimise sugar cravings – especially if having a little bit will intensify your craving for chocolate bars or sweets. That will make things much harder. If you find that having a diet soft drink has this effect on you, the recommendation is to try and limit it. But if you don't have this effect, diet soft drink and artificial sugar can be a helpful stepping stone for slowly reducing your sugar intake in the long term without consuming the calories that come with straight sugar. If it makes you feel like you had a snack and you feel satisfied, and this helps you stick to your calorie budget and keeps you away from high-calorie sugary foods, this is a good thing. It's really individual.'

## No need to stress, sweetheart – we've done all the counting for you!

Although it's really important that you have some understanding of the big picture of what's good for you nutritionally speaking, it can get a tad overwhelming, can't it? This is why we have dedicated the second half of this book to meal plans and fabulously yummy, nutritionally balanced recipes to take the hard work away for you. Easy peasy, lemon squeezy!

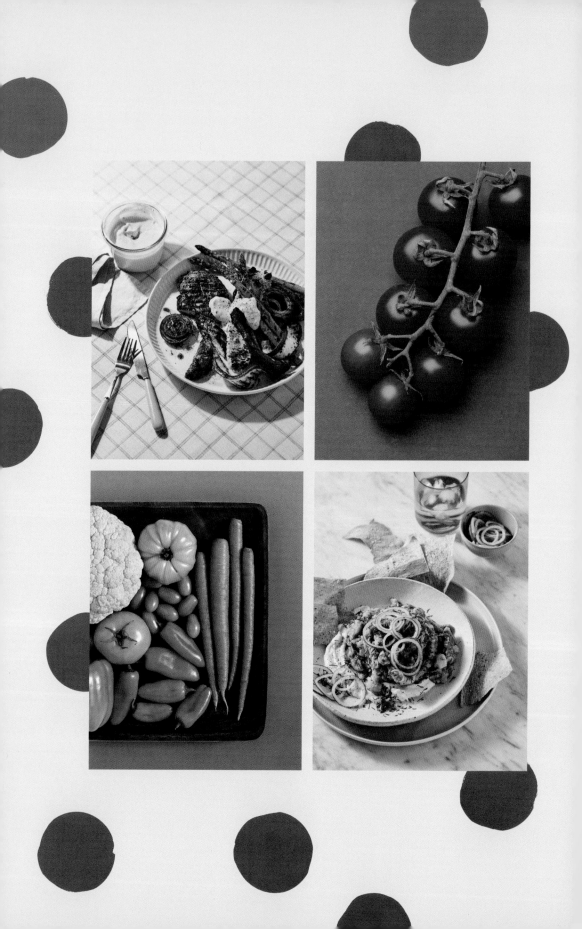

# CHAPTER

# 5

# The forever solution

# Your new healthy life

One of the major pitfalls of traditional diets is that they don't provide you with a plan for maintaining it long-term. You go 'on' a diet then 'off' a diet so there's no guidance for transitioning into real life. This is what usually causes people to slip back into unhealthy habits and put the weight they lost back on. That's. Not. Us.

Intermittent fasting (IF) isn't really a diet at all; it's a lifestyle, which means it's *meant* to be practised long-term – hence all the variable methods. It's designed for wherever you're up to on your weight-loss journey, and, once you've lost the kilos, for easily maintaining your goal weight for good.

Which brings us to this next chapter @ the four-week mark. This is actually an exciting time, because after you've completed four weeks of IF you've achieved an incredible amount!

- You've heard Dr Krista's explanation of how it all works and read her amazing new findings.
- You've tried our three fave methods and likely have an idea of which one works best for you right now.
- You've even tried supercharging and now know our secret to losing weight even faster!
- PLUS you've got your head around everything food-related: how to be a dirty faster and still lose weight, calorie counting (or not), eating for fullness and nutrition, portion sizes, sugar …

… wow. You've come a long way, baby!

Now it's time to step off the four-week roadmap and into the next phase of your new, healthy fasting life which we call The Forever Solution.

## Welcome to week five and beyond

So, how did your first four weeks go? Did you float through each week like a breeze? Were some methods easier than others? Did you have the odd faceplant into cheesecake and/or pizza, then shrug it off and move your fast day? To all of that, we say congratulations! You've got your head around things now and maybe you've dropped a couple of kilos too, right?

Woohoo – take a bow!

And it's also time to take stock. At the very beginning you took steps to really understand your starting point. The same should happen here as you start the next part of your journey. Time to whip out a pen and paper – we're going to take a good look back so that we can propel you forward!

*Remember: IF is a lifestyle, not a fad diet. And supercharging is here to stay!*

## Step 1:

### HERE'S WHERE YOU GET TO PICK A METHOD … FOR NOW

We say 'for now' because this can be a tricky decision, but take the pressure off. Swapping methods around is as easy as ditching the jeans and popping on a skirt just before you walk out the door because the SFD lifestyle is super flexy, remember? You make it work for you, not the other way around. So, this could be a good time to jot down a comparison list of which one suited your lifestyle best, or perhaps you don't need to and you already know which one you want to continue with.

Ideally, you'll pick a method that will take you to your next goal/milestone and review it again when you get there, but not to worry if you change your mind along the way.

## Step 2:

### TAKE NOTE OF WHAT TRICKS WORK FOR *YOU*

Think back to anything that made fasting easier. It could have been a recipe, a distraction, a hunger-staving snack, a new habit or dirty-fasting hack (see page 57). Keep these personalised crutches front of mind (perhaps as part of your daily list?) to help you stay the course in the future.

## Step 3:

### GOALS AND MILESTONES

Time to go back to the Six C Cycle (see page 58) to set a new milestone and get focused on your short-term and long-term goals. This includes taking measurements again to see how much they've gone down already (!), weighing yourself (likewise!), choosing a piece of clothing you want to wear and hanging it at the front of the wardrobe … you know, incredibly awesome, motivating stuff like that. Four weeks ago was so four weeks ago! This progress checkpoint activity is going to become one of your favourite parts of the journey as you get closer and closer to reaching your big goal.

## Step 4:

### THE TORTOISE AND THE HARE

Just a little word on expectation before we move on: The Fastest Diet is the fastest diet for you. If you did exceed expectations and smash your goals – hooray! But if you only lost a little (or maybe with a few hiccups along the way or none at all) – be kind to yourself. Some people will take to fasting much easier and lose weight faster. And some people are known affectionately as 'Fast Turtles', but remember who won the race? We've had a lot of readers/members who've been slow and steady in their weight loss but have got to goal and never looked back. Progress is progress – keep your eyes on the scales prize!

## How to have your cake and eat it, too (aka, fast and have fun!)

IF is all about the forever solution. The whole point is to integrate your fasting habits with your fab life and never feel like you're on a diet – otherwise, it will be too hard to stick to. So, to the fun bits!

### EAT, DRINK AND BE MERRY BECAUSE TOMORROW YOU CAN ALWAYS FAST

Can you think of the last time you were at a party or event and there was no food/drink temptation? Unless it was some super boring political 'party' speech or something equally dreary, we're betting no. Eating and drinking is entwined in our social culture, so our plan is to always plan to include it. (No wonder socialisers love SFD.) Obviously, timing-wise, we always recommend planning your fasting schedule around social events so you can enjoy yourself totally guilt-free.

Having said that, why not lower the calories as a matter of course? Some of these socialising hacks really work for us and we barely even notice them, they've become so habitual:

- If you're attending a bring-a-plate party or barbecue, make sure it's one of our fabulous salads or dishes in this book and revel in the praise. #shucksitwasnothing
- Make sure you drink plenty of water so that you're hydrated (and satiated). We do the glass of water for every glass of wine rule, which is totally easy to stick to.
- Eat a healthy snack beforehand so that you're not super hungry and tempted to attack the bread basket/scoff all the deep-fried hors d'oeuvres.
- Many restaurant portions are much larger than they need to be. Don't be afraid to ask if anyone is up for sharing a main, side or dessert. Sometimes an entrée is generous enough to be a main, too. Sneak a peek at the other tables to gauge this. Why waste money on a meal you can't finish or, worse still, force yourself to finish and sit with a protesting pudding stomach half the night? After all, you need to leave some room for champagne or dessert.
- Studies show that people tend to consume more calories in social situations often because they're distracted (oh look – shiny disco ball) or nervous (uh-oh, what's this guy's name again?) or just plain excited (woohoo – I'm out! Must do everything!). Whatever the reason, you adopt a more relaxed approach to your food/drink consumption and may not really be aware of how much you're shovelling/guzzling. If this is you, try mindful eating: slow down, pay attention and really enjoy it.

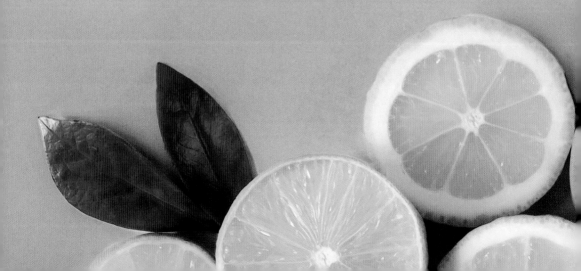

# Myles

**LOST** 30 kg

Size 42 to size 36

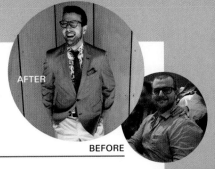

AFTER

BEFORE

Twenty-nine-year-old Myles has a demanding career in the media, but it does have its perks, including a very social side to the business. As much as Myles loves this part of his job, it was playing havoc with his weight, especially as he also enjoys his social life with his friends on the weekends. Intermittent fasting was the perfect solution and has suited Myles's social and personal lifestyle to a T.

Myles says intermittent fasting has become the perfect way for him to enjoy his social life while maintaining a healthy weight: 'Going out to lunches and dinners with clients and industry associates are some of my favourite things-to-do. I also really enjoy having lots of fun with my friends so my life revolves around gourmet food and cheeky bevvies.'

Unfortunately Myles was paying the price on the scales for all of this socialising, with his weight tipping 122 kg. He knew he had to find a way to get things back under control.'What attracted me to intermittent fasting was the fact that I only had to be "good" for three days a week and I could still wine and dine on the other four days – albeit trying to be a little healthier as well. Once I learned how much food you could have for your fast days when you made good choices (like lots of vegies, salads, high-quality proteins and clever foods like cauliflower rice) I found it wasn't too hard. Then I could eat, drink and be merry the following day if I wanted.

'Eating within an 8-hour window has become a lifestyle for me. This means I indulge without any guilt on weekends (and trust me I do let my hair down), knowing I can pop in some fast days during the week to balance it all out.'

The weight quickly fell away and Myles lost a staggering 30 kg. He went from 122 kg to 92 kg and has kept it off successfully for two years.'Since dropping 30 kilos I am so much fitter! I am also way more confident and love dressing up to go out. Additionally, I love to move my body and have gotten involved in boxing and weight training, which I would never have been motivated to do before.After many years of struggling with my weight, I feel like I've finally nailed it. Life is awesome!'

**'Eating within an 8-hour window has become a lifestyle for me. This means I indulge without any guilt on weekends (and trust me I do let my hair down) knowing I can pop in some fast days during the week to balance it all out.'**

## WHAT ABOUT BUBBLY?

Our recommendation is to follow the expert recommendation. The National Health and Medical Research Council of Australia suggests no more than 10 standard drinks per week and no more than four standard drinks in a day. This is to mitigate health risks associated with drinking alcohol, like liver damage and high blood pressure among many other things.

When it comes to weight management, alcohol is unfortunately the bad guy again. Alcohol comes in at 7 calories per gram. In our minds, this is probably worse than fat because alcohol doesn't come with any nutrients like good fats do. Worse still, because alcohol is a toxin, your liver will work hard to deal with it and hold off processing any other calories that you've had (beer nuts, juice or mixers).

On fast days, we don't recommend consuming alcohol because we don't think that the empty calories are worth it. On normal days, however, you're welcome to sip as you wish! On top of the recommended consumption for health, we would also suggest opting for wine, champagne, beer or spirits served neat or with soda water as opposed to sugary mixers, syrups or cocktails. If you feel like something fancy, look for drinks made with muddled fruits, tea or steeped fruit for flavour. Or ask the bartender if you can have a splash of syrup instead of a full shot. Sweet.

*Eat, drink and be merry for tomorrow we fast!*

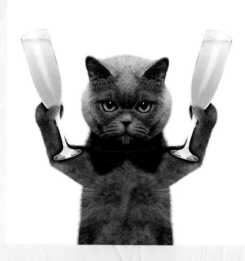

## Cheers to our favourite low-calorie drinks!

- Vodka, fresh lime and soda – 70 calories
- Gin, fresh lime, rose water and cucumber – 75 calories
- Spiced rum, diet ginger beer, fresh ginger and lime juice – 81 calories
- Champagne and dry white wine – 100 calories
- Low-carb and low-alcohol beer – between 55 and 100 calories, depending on the brand
- 1 part Moscato with 1 part soda sparkling water – 65 calories per 150 ml
- Sparkling mineral water and fresh lime – zero calories, zero hangover, zero taboo!

## Did someone say dessert?

The awesome SFD news is there's always room for dessert and you'll still lose weight on The Fastest Diet. Mind you, there are ways to keep the calories a bit lower if you've used up quite a few on other things today. This could be sharing a dessert if you're out for a meal or getting the smaller size on offer if you're just having a treat. Another idea is just to taste it so you don't feel like you're missing out on the experience, or to keep the hostess or host at the dinner party satisfied after their hours of work in the kitchen.

Having said all that, if you've got plenty of cal wiggle room (and you do on a non-fast day), indulge away!

At home, we like to try and focus on DIY desserts because you get to choose what you add in. Two of our NEW faves to make are Strawberry Coco Froyo, sweetened with honey and real strawberries – 99 calories per serve (page 216) and Chocolate Crackle Bites with no added sugar – 101 calories per serve (page 215).

### FLEX THE FLEXXY FACTOR

The great thing about trying all the different methods is not only knowing how to do them, but you can also see how they might suit different weeks of your life and plan accordingly. Each method is adaptable and can be used as needed. Or just because you like to mix things up. #foreversolution

Here are some examples of how you can flex for life:

- **On holidays.** Use the part-day method with a more relaxed eating window (say 10 hours rather than eight). Basically, just sleep in and skip the breakfast buffet. Or not. You can always do a supercharge when you get home instead.
- **Festive season.** Fast on non-party days, feast on the others. This will really suit the 2-day or 3-day methods. That way you can manage your calendar rather than your socialising. (Ain't no one putting baby in a party 'diet corner'.)
- **Stressed or super-busy.** For times when you have a lot on your mind, the last thing you need is to cloud it with complicated food choices or stress eat and make everything worse by gaining weight. When life gets particularly challenging, we turn our fasting focus down by using the part-day method and having less food planning to think about. This also allows us windows where we can have some food comfort, aka stay calm and have a hot chocolate. #becauseyoucan

# Shanna

**LOST** 16 kg

Size 18 to size 12

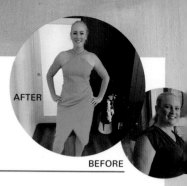

AFTER

BEFORE

Shanna says that for years she's portrayed herself as a positive person but pretending to be okay and confident all the time was exhausting, especially after putting on weight. No matter what she tried, she always regained it back. Then she adapted all three methods of SFD into her life and reclaimed her truly happy, confident self.

'For years I've presented myself as this confident, happy and carefree person,' Shanna admits, 'but in all honesty, that couldn't have been further from the truth. On the inside I was struggling with low self-esteem, self-doubt, self-criticism and a severe lack of self-worth. I was suffering from depression and battling ongoing health issues. I was losing interest in social activities, snapping at my loved ones for no reason … I was irritable and losing my sense of humour and fun. In truth, I was losing the last little bits of myself that made me ME!

'For as long as I can remember, I've struggled to maintain my weight. I've tried shake diets, detox diets, restricted calorie diets, gym prescribed meal plans and even doctor prescribed medication and injections. None of the diets, eating plans or strict exercise regimes I tried were sustainable for me long-term. I felt stuck and hopeless. I'd become resigned to the fact that I would never be the truly confident, energetic and fun person I used to be. Then my beautiful aunt had great success with SFD, losing over 20 kg in less than a year, so I took the plunge and signed up, still sceptical that it would be another short-lived attempt but, as it turned out, it was easy and maintainable.

'The biggest difference was definitely how flexible it was. It was so refreshing to find a program that fit in with my busy life instead of having to change my life to fit the diet. Having the three different methods to choose from meant I could quickly and easily adapt my diet to suit my busy mum/work life, make allowances for social events and prepare food within my cooking capabilities. To date I have lost just over 16 kg, and I've achieved all of this while also dealing with depression and ongoing health issues. It's given me my life back. I've rediscovered the energy and zest that I thought I'd lost forever. I'm no longer a spectator, watching the world carry on around me. SFD has helped me to reclaim my truly happy, confident self and continues to change my life in ways I didn't think possible.'

**'Having the three different methods to choose from meant I could quickly and easily adapt my diet to suit my busy mum/work life … It's given me my life back.'**

# Female fasting fallacies

As women, we go through so many biological shifts in life it's often hard to predict if today will be fine and dandy ... or bloaty, weepy, flushy and crampy. Some people might see those shifts as reasons to rule out fasting because it might make things harder, but the opposite is actually true.

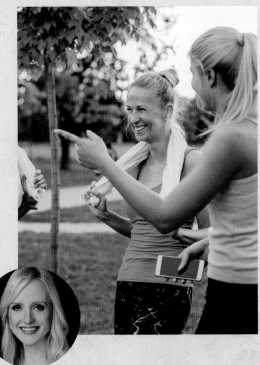

As most women-of-a-certain-age know all too well, our bodies change as we get older, and fasting actually helps us manage some of those changes, especially during menopause. We asked **Megan Ramos**, a clinical educator and expert on therapeutic fasting and low-carbohydrate diets, to weigh-in on this all-important topic. Megan has guided more than 14,000 people through their weight-loss journeys and is highly qualified to dispel any fallacies littering the hormone trail. Here's what she had to say about a few common fallacies.

## FALLACY #1

### FASTING IS BAD FOR FERTILITY

Spoiler alert: it's absolutely not.

Megan says: 'Being in a healthy weight range is important for fertility. As is treating PCOS and insulin resistance – you have to treat these things first – and fasting is a great way to do that. We treat them in the same way that we would treat people with diabetes, post-menopausal women or men, and that is with the goal of lowering insulin resistance. Once the insulin issues are resolved, then we start to optimise fasting for fertility.'

#HUGEfemalefastingwin

## FALLACY #2

### FASTING IS NOT SAFE FOR WOMEN

Pfft. Over to Megan.

'We've seen over 20,000 people and over 70 per cent of the people that we work with (in the clinic or online) are women who span all ages of adulthood. The most important thing to remember is that we're treating insulin resistance – once that is reversed, everything else falls into place. I've only seen IF give women back control of their health, their waistlines and their metabolic health (like reversing their diabetes). Clinically there's no reason why there is this fear. Don't be afraid to try it: it can change your life like it changed mine.'

## I'LL NEVER BE ABLE TO FAST DURING MY PERIOD BECAUSE I GET RAVENOUS

To answer this, Megan starts by explaining our hormonal stages:

'We really look at females in two different hormonal phases in adult life: you have women who are menstruating and you have women that are in that menopause transition or postmenopausal phase. There are very different hormonal profiles, and that definitely is impacted by fasting,' says Megan.

'Women experience different hormonal fluctuations throughout the monthly cycle. In the first half of our cycle – we call that the follicular phase – we produce follicles and one of those follicles will grow to become dominant and release an egg at ovulation. Once that egg is released, we enter the luteal phase of our cycle. These two different phases are dominated by different hormones that can really affect hunger.'

*So is one phase easier than the other? Turns out the answer to that is yes!*

'During the follicular phase, oestrogen is dominant,' Megan explains. 'Our ovaries produce a form of oestrogen called oestradiol that generally improves mood and suppresses appetite. During the first half of the cycle, women feel like they could fast forever – it feels easy and effortless.'

*Sounds perfect! But what about that second phase …?*

'During the luteal phase, progesterone is the dominant hormone and testosterone rises a bit as well. Progesterone is an appetite-stimulating hormone. So, during the second half of the cycle, our appetites are running high hormonally. This is because ovulation has happened and our bodies are getting ready to nurture a potential embryo. Especially around day 21, when progesterone is elevated, we're so enticed to eat.'

*So how can fasting still work?*

'During the second half of the cycle, we focus on time-restricted eating, shorter intermittent fasts, or simply nutrients and food. Menstruation doesn't always fit that classic 28-day cycle, so you've got to go with the ebbs and flows of how a person is feeling. If they feel like they could really fast and it feels really easy, then that's a good sign. If they feel like fasting is like trying to run up an escalator that's moving, then we focus on time-restricted eating. Embrace your cycle and let these hormonal shifts dictate your pattern.'

*And it gets easier over time, right?*

'What we find is that three or four months down the road, it does become a little bit less difficult. The cravings are not intense, the appetite is not as wild.'

*And of course, you feel much more energetic and able to handle your periods when you are carrying less weight. #femalefastingwin*

## FALLACY #4

### FASTING WILL MESS MY CYCLES UP

'If a woman starts with a regular 28-day cycle, during those first four to six months, they can have some irregularities. With weight loss, there are major hormonal shifts that are happening in the body, and it can throw the cycle off. Most of the time, it resolves within three periods, but sometimes it can take up to six months.'

*Although not always ...*

'The opposite can also happen! If someone comes into the fast with something like polycystic ovarian syndrome (PCOS) where they're having irregular cycles, they will likely still remain irregular for about four to six months. After that, then we start to experience more regularity.'

*Fasting as a period regulator? Wow. #anotherfemalefastingwin*

## FALLACY #5

### MENOPAUSE IS TOO MUCH OF A HOT MESS, FASTING WILL MAKE IT WORSE

*First things first:*

'Menopause is a big hot mess that can lead to weight gain and low moods.'

*But Megan says weight issues can start long before that.*

'Before that, during perimenopause, we transition into oestrogen dominance, which can contribute to weight gain. Then during menopause, the production of appetite-suppressing oestradiol starts to slow. It gets replaced by its awful step-sister, estrone" which encourages the body to hold onto fat.'

*Eep! But it gets better, right?*

'Post-menopause, you also produce less testosterone, which can help burn fat. There is just a tonne of hormonal shifts that happen. It will level out hormonally, but then you have this excess weight.'

*Enter fasting? You betcha.*

'At the start, weight loss can be a little bit sluggish. But what we see is if they stick with it, with the understanding that they're not broken, and that their system might require more of a tune-up, and if they adhere to their fasting practice – at around six weeks, the weight loss starts to pick up.'

*Hooray! #olderfemalefastingwin (We so deserve some good news after all that!)*

## ... but what about hunger?

When we talk to people that haven't heard of IF they'll usually ask (in one way or another), 'But aren't you hungry?'

It seems a funny question when you consider that traditional diets leave you feeling starving most of the time as you try to survive on boring salads, and our way of life embraces regular feasting – but we digress.

Are we hungry? Yes, sometimes we are, of course; however, periods without food doesn't automatically mean periods of hunger. That's like asking someone if they're hungry while they're asleep.

Hunger's a funny thing, too. For a start, it alters once you get used to fasting. Hunger is a physiological sensation that tells your body it's time to eat. If you're used to eating all the time, you'll be hungry because your body is expecting food – but it doesn't mean that it needs food right at that moment. It's just a habit. The Hunger Habit, as we often call it. When your body gets used to delayed eating or having lower-calorie days, the hunger adjusts to what the body expects. For example, on a part-day fast, if your usual eating window is between 12 pm and 8 pm, you'll start finding that you get hungry around 11:30ish. Amazing, really. The body has formed a new habit – the Fasting Habit.

There are two important hormonal players in the hunger games of your body: ghrelin and leptin.

Ghrelin is an appetite stimulant (think the little gremlin that makes you feel hungry) but it's essentially just a signal. It's not really telling you anything important either – your body is used to getting food, and ghrelin is just wondering where that food is. Clever you knows that food will come as per your fasting schedule, so you're totally fine with overriding the ghrelin hunger signal and letting it pass. Studies also show that ghrelin tends to increase after weight loss, and scientists think it's because your body is trying to get you back to your previous weight. This does wear off as your body adjusts though, so don't worry.

Leptin does the opposite to ghrelin in that it makes you feel satiated. Interestingly, research shows that people with obesity tend to have more leptin circulating in their body, but it doesn't have the proper appetite-suppressing effect because they may have developed leptin-resistance.

Science also proves that this applies to all weight-loss methods, so it's not true that fasting makes you hungrier (see, not just our boring salad theory here). One study compared the appetites of participants that were IF and those on traditional diets (continuous calorie reduction) and found no significant differences in appetite – even after a fast day. Ha! Your body isn't being mean ... it's just used to functioning under certain energy balance conditions. It likes routine, but you can teach the ol' bod new tricks.

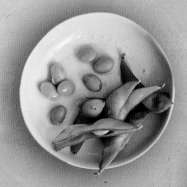
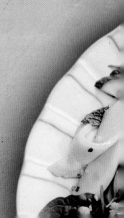

## HUNGER SHM-UNGER

Some people let hunger build up in their minds as this big thing they will need to overcome and deal with but as we say and pinky-promise, you will get used to it. And it will fade. A lot of experienced fasters actually say they welcome hunger as they know they are in the fat-burning zone (ketosis) – i.e. the fat cells are breaking down, baby! You also know that feasting is on the way and how good does food taste when you've got an appetite?!

Aside from that, once you've overcome hunger a few times you'll know that it's totally doable and it might even feel – *gasp* – easy. Until then, here are some handy hacks to help you hold out until your fast is finished:

- Drink water! Hydration is a satiety signal, remember? A lot of the time people think they're hungry, but they're actually thirsty. We can't emphasise enough how true we've found this to be! So, yes, quench your thirst first.
- Um ... is it hunger, or is it appetite? Hunger is physiological, i.e. tummy grumbles. Appetite is a desire to eat influenced by a bunch of non-biological things like boredom, habit, environment, emotions, that stupid ad on TV with the cheesy crust pizza. If you're getting signals from your appetite, change something to make it easier to satiate that. For example, if you're bored, call a friend!
- Lean on a dirty-fasting crutch like tea or bone broth or some strawberries to make it easier (see page 57).

## Other healthy habits

While you can absolutely lose weight with IF alone, we have to make honourable mentions to a few other healthy habits. Not only will they support your IF efforts, but they'll make you shinier, peppier and healthier all round!

### LET'S GET PHYSICAL!

Movement promotes health in sooooo many ways. It burns calories, keeps you limber, often improves your mood, strengthens muscles, prevents ageing issues (e.g. osteoporosis) and it can keep your cardiovascular system healthy, too. When we were cave-people, we moved all the time! (Those pesky wolf packs kept us on our prehistoric toes.)

These days, most of us live sans life-and-death hunting expeditions and have fairly sedentary lives. Almost half of working women describe their days as 'mostly sitting' (!). The good news is that we don't really have to do that much exercise to get to a healthy level. It's recommended that 20+ minutes of moderate exercise each day, with some strength and toning twice a week thrown in, will do the trick. Strength training is important, especially for older women, as it minimises the risk of falls and broken bones. Unfortunately, less than 25 per cent of people meet daily movement needs.

If you want to join the healthy percentile club, you can do so pretty easily, and you don't need to join an actual fitness club to do it. You just need to start to add more movement to your day. This can be a walk, a spot of yoga, chasing your dog, pilates or dancing around while you do the dishes. Do whatever makes movement fun, and you might find that once you start, you'll get your groove on and there'll be no stopping you. Vacuum boogieing, anyone?

Our absolute fave exercise is to go for a super relaxed walk in the early morning and/ or after dinner. It's a nice way to relax, think,

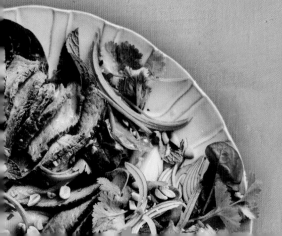

and get some alone time or time with a friend or loved one. A 2022 study found that a light walk anywhere from 2–20 minutes after a meal helped to process glucose and insulin, especially compared to sitting after a meal. If you do this after your last meal in the day, it may help your body switch to a fasting state – faster!

Just one more point (before you walk away because we're still banging on about walking): it's actually good for more than just the body, it's good for the mind and your spirit.

Physically, it's great for all the reasons outlined above, naturally, but things are going on mentally too. It frees the mind as you process all that busyness upstairs and the body releases endorphins that make you feel happier. As for your spirit? Well, not to get too hippy or anything, but all that focus on nature does calm you on a deeper level. Breathe ...

---

SFD has been a life-changer for me. I have arthritis everywhere in my body and also irritable bowel disease, which is very debilitating. Since I started, I have lost 8 kg, gone from a size 14/16 down to a size 10/12. I can now walk 18,000 steps everyday no problem. My health has improved so much, I feel 20 years younger and the best is being able to run around with my grandsons. Thank you so much Vic + Gen – you saved my life!

LIZZIE WILSON

## AHHHH ... SLEEP

Turns out that most of us are pretty good at getting our Zs when it comes to the amount we sleep per night, with a reported average of 7–8 hours. On the face of it, this is good news, as getting adequate amounts of sleep is crucial for supporting metabolism, endocrine/cardiovascular health, mood and immunity.

However, if you're reading this and starting to mutter 'but I ...' you're probably already guessing that statistic doesn't quite give the whole picture. Getting that much sleep in theory is one thing, but *quality of sleep* is a whole other issue.

If you struggle with a sleep problem, like sleep apnoea, or insomnia, or sleep for short stints interspersed by staring at the ceiling and trying to count sheep, you're not alone. Almost 50 per cent of people report having at least two sleep-related issues. It's worth improving your sleep, not only for general health, but for weight loss, too.

Scientists have found an association between short sleep duration and an increase in ghrelin (the hungry hormone). Another study in overweight adults that slept less than 6.5 hours tested the effect of sleep extension. They found that extending sleep by just 1.5 hours a night resulted in significant decreases in energy intake – 270 calories less than the control group!

Yep, more sleeping less sheeping will help you to lose weight. So how to improve things?

Getting more sleep can be a frustrating business. Sometimes it seems almost impossible to get back to the land of nod, to the point you start to wonder, 'How do I do this again?' Such thoughts are actually futile, because of course sleeping isn't something you can just 'do' on mental command. In fact, you need to trick your conscious mind into relinquishing control and letting the body and the subconscious mind take over. Here are a few zzz tips.

- Make sure you spend lots of time in sunlight or under lights during the day (so your body acknowledges it's awake), then really turn the lights down at night (we like switching from overhead lights to moody lights/candles after dinner).
- Don't lie there swiping away on your phone. Bed is for sleeping, not entertainment (unless special cuddles are in order ...which will also help you to sleep afterwards ... ahem).
- No caffeine before bedtime and not too much alcohol. (We don't care how much fun special cuddles might be after an overly generous tipple. You'll regret it when it wears off at 3 am and it's back to just you and the sheep.)
- Exercise daily as this will improve your sleep quality and duration as well as your alertness during the day.
- Try to go to bed at the same time and get up at the same time.
- Do something relaxing as bedtime approaches like a skin routine or taking a leisurely bath.
- Avoid napping during the day.
- Manage worries by jotting them down before you go to bed and setting them aside lest those sheep turn into bills, work issues, things you don't want to forget to do etc. etc.
- Meditate by relaxing each part of your body one by one and breathing deeply, emptying your mind. #ommmmzzzzzzz

## SNACKY FACTS

We all love a nice snack. Problem is, constant grazing could be the cause of constant cravings.

Additionally, the portions are small and are unlikely to stretch your stomach enough to send satiety signals to the brain. This could be why you feel hungry shortly after. If you're used to lots of small snacks during the day, don't go cold turkey. Instead, eat a variety of snacks that include protein (like turkey!) and healthy fats (e.g. avocado, nuts) to help stimulate the other satiety signals.

It's a great idea to have a small healthy snack just prior to a meal if you are super hungry – especially on a fast day – as it takes the edge off your hunger and you feel fuller earlier (remember it takes 20 minutes for your brain to register that your tummy is delightfully full). It's all about timing on a part-time diet! Not denying.

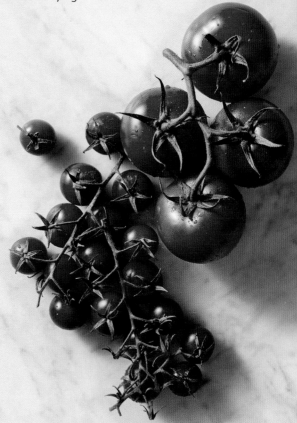

## #fastfails

'Hello, I'm perfect,' said no one, ever. You will have accidental fast fails. You will accidentally face-plant into a tub of ice-cream! You will open the door to your BFF holding champagne and takeout and say, 'Alrigghttty, then!'

Fortunately, we are so anti-diet here at SFD, we want you to #fastfail because we want you to be happy and live a normal life!

Here's why it does ... not ... matter. And is in fact, a good thing.

**1** **It's your SFD prerogative to change your mind!** Failing at doing a fasting day only goes to show you how flexible this is. You can simply make tomorrow a fast day instead.

**2** **It makes you happy to indulge.** No one is going to stick to a diet they hate long term, or if they do they'll be miserable a lot of the time. #fastfails will help you to keep on going with a smile because yay – spontaneous fun!

**3** **You get to have fun with all the non-diet people out there** – because you're one of them, even as you are, in fact, losing weight. You're not a boring 'on-a-diet' person – you're vibing a forever solution, you super faster you. #lovethisWOL

## But what if it all suddenly ... um, stops

Look, up in the sky, it's a bird, it's a plane, it's ... a wall.

Eeep. It happens. Sometimes IF does suddenly seem to just stop working and you hit a plateau. But before you kick the scales to the corner and storm off to the fridge in disgust, you need to know a few very important reasons why this might have happened and what you can do to get straight back on the fast track.

## Step 1:

### IS IT SOMETHING ... OBVIOUS?

Are you really sticking to it? Hey, it's just us, living inside the pages of this book. You can be honest here. Studies show that most reported plateaus at six to eight months occur because people get a bit lackadaisical.

This doesn't mean you've done it on purpose or have done anything wrong. It could just be that you're out of your fasting 'honeymoon period'. It's just like at the start of an exciting new relationship: you're dressing up and kind of obsessed, but after a few months you're happy to have date nights on the couch in your trackies. At the beginning of your fasting journey, you would have been super diligent and it's normal for you to start to relax and maybe over-flex, especially if you've already lost some weight.

If this sounds like you, note to self: this is actually a good thing. You're comfortable with IF now. It's part of your life. But it does sound like it might be time to up your game and recommit.

So, let's assess this for what it truly is:

1. Are you exactly keeping to the hours/days of your method?
2. Are you 100 per cent confident that you're eating the right amount of calories or are you guessing a fair bit?

Fasting doesn't have a lot of rules but those two main ones are really important. If you're not sticking to them that's okay, you can just tighten things up a little starting tomorrow. We guarantee the scales will start moving again when you do.

# Step 2:

## IF YOU'VE LOST A LOT OF WEIGHT, CHECK YOUR TDEE AGAIN

Well, this is kind of a nice problem to have right? It's always a good idea to check that you're still eating the right number of calories per day. And if you've lost a lot of weight (woohoo – go you), your calorie needs will have gone down – so it's a good idea to recalculate your TDEE (see page 59) to make sure your goal posts are correct. No biggie really, you just don't need quite as much food anymore and your appetite likely reflects that. If not, just start swapping out a few lower-calorie meals or snacks to bring it back in line with your new TDEE.

# Step 3:

## DO YOU NEED TO GET DOWN OR GET LESS DIRTY …?

If you're fasting by the book it may be time to cheat. Hey, you played nice, time to trick that body into blasting through this wall and flying across this plateau to fasting happyland once more. Here's a few sneaky tricks to get things moving:

**Get down:** Is it time to fiddle with the numbers a tad? For example, if you chose the 2-day or 3-day method, try throwing in an extra fast day. If you are doing the part-day method, perhaps you could extend your fasting window by an hour or two?

**Get less dirty**: If you were dirty fasting, maybe you could try clean fasting (see page 57). It's funny how little differences can make big differences at this stage and you know you can always go back to your dirty ways once this wall is out of the way. Your body just needs a little reassurance that you're also committed right now, is all. If you were fairly loose about nutrition, maybe you could try paying closer attention to how much processed food, alcohol and sugar you consume.

**Supercharge it.** Drumroll please, because this is one of the best ways to get through a plateau of all, The Fastest Diet BIG point of difference: the supercharging method (see page 28). It has been the game-changer at this stage for so many of our readers/members and we highly recommend you take the reins, blow your own trumpet and … charge! #smashingthrough

# Step 4:

## IT'S NOT YOU IT'S … EVERYTHING ELSE

~~~~~~~~~~~~~~~~~~~~~~~~~~~~~~~~

Maybe this is actually nothing to do with fasting at all. What we eat and drink can be very much circumstantial. If something/ someone else is disrupting your fasting success, you need to focus on resolving that issue rather than trying to force yourself onto a stricter regimen.

If you're stressed and that's causing you to overeat, could you start meditating or go for more walks? If you overeat when you're bored, could you find a new hobby? If you find that you let loose a bit too much in social situations, could you try one of our social hacks? These situations are all influenced by a bunch of things – habits, social life, people, emotions – that can't be overcome by a sheer will to not eat or eat less. Forget about it. First, try to find non-food related solutions that will make it easier for you. Then get back to fasting.

Kindness note: If you're going through something really difficult, allow yourself time to go through it. Maybe you can use some more fasting crutches during this tricky period and accept that weight loss can be a little slower until you find your feet again. Life can be hard. And you're only human. Always remember to be kind to you, first and foremost.

# Step 5:

## ARE YOU … THERE YET?

~~~~~~~~~~~~~~~~~~~~~~~~~~~~~~~~

Another reason you might have hit a plateau is that – get ready for it – you could be at a healthy weight! If you're within a healthy BMI range already, take a pause to think about whether you need to lose more weight. If the lofty goal you set at the start was lower than what you weigh now it might be worth considering why you set that goal.

Is it realistic? Are you really a curvaceous Sophia Loren aiming for an Audrey Hepburn body? Should you instead aim for more tone, rather than skinny? If you're within a healthy weight range and still want to see changes in your physique, it could be a good time to shift your focus to exercise and use IF as a tool for maintenance instead.

Yes, we just used the word 'maintenance'. If you find you actually are at your goal, it's time to move into the next stage with your head held high. You did it. You made it. Welcome to your happier, healthier life, you super faster, you!

*Be kind to yourself, you are doing the best you can.*

# Michelle

**LOST** 60 kg

Size 28
to size 14

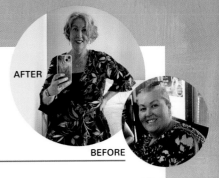

AFTER

BEFORE

Before finding SFD Michelle tipped the scales at 147 kg and, with major health issues, she was getting desperate to shed weight, but she was 'lost'. SFD has turned her life around. Michelle says she's never going back and has no doubt she'll reach her final goal, maintaining this for the rest of her life.

'Before finding SFD my weight gain had got out of control,' Michelle says. 'I believed there was no way I was going to get a hold on this. I was having to buy larger sizes each time I went shopping. At a size 28, the only pants that would fit me were leggings. Being diagnosed with melanoma in 2020, I needed to fly to my specialist every three months. I dreaded these flights, being too big for the seats. I had to ask for a seat extender every time I boarded. I was embarrassed, struggling to do everyday tasks without exhaustion.' Michelle tried everything she could to lose the weight and was even considering lap band surgery, which she never believed in or liked the idea of, 'but I was desperate'.

'Before SFD I was lost. I was giving up hope but then I saw SFD on TV and decided to commit to a 28-day challenge.' Michelle started with doing the 3-day method, saying, 'I liked that you have the flexibility of changing your fast days over if you have an unplanned blowout. The program, along with my coach Emma, soon showed me it isn't just about diet, this lifestyle change also requires a mindset adjustment and wow, has my life changed as a result! From a starting weight of 147 kg, to date I have lost 60 kg. Going from a size 28 to a size 14 means I can now shop confidently in 'normal' fashion shops rather than going to the Plus Size section in variety stores.

'I know that I'll reach my goal weight and from there I'll have the confidence to maintain this for the rest of my life. I love that I can enjoy myself to the fullest at dinner parties, holidays – in fact, every day. I will never see that "big" mean-to-myself girl in the mirror ever again. I have learnt to love who I am, to be kinder to myself and therefore kinder to everyone else. Most of all, it taught me #noguilt. I see now I was a spectator and I am never going to be that again. I have changed careers and I am living life to its fullest. If anyone is unsure, if they are looking down that tunnel and only seeing darkness, believe me when I tell you there is light and it is the SFD way. '

**'I have learnt to love who I am, to be kinder to myself and therefore kinder to everyone else. Most of all, it taught me #noguilt.'**

## Don't throw in the towel

Hands up if you've ever had a couple of salt and vinegar chips, then thought, 'Oh well, I've broken the diet now. May as well eat the whole party bag ...'?

Yep. Totally relate. Up until we started IF, that was our thought process, too. That's the problem with the whole going on/going off a diet paradigm: it's broken. Literally. If you scoff the chips, you throw in the towel because you think, 'There's no point now – may as well eat a tub of ice-cream too.'

But oh, how different it is on a part-time diet. Eating those chips doesn't break a single thing, nor does it degenerate into a gorging session inside the freezer, because you are safe in the knowledge that all is not lost and you can just swap your fast day to tomorrow.

The only towel you'll be throwing is a beach towel in the car because you'll no longer be afraid to bare your body on the sand. #nomorebingeingsadness

*Remember, the trick is to find what works for you long-term.*

## 24-hour fast reset

Okay so you've heard of it ... it sounds a little scary ... but guess what? The 24-hour fast reset is totally doable once you're used to fasting, especially once you nail part-day and supercharging!

**WHY DO IT?**
Well, if you're feeling like you've fallen off the wagon (e.g. been on a tour of Swiss chocolate factories ... or just a tour of your pantry post-Easter), this is a great way to up your motivation and likely get a quick win on the scales before zooming back into your usual method!

**HOW DO I DO IT?**
To hit the reset switch, all you have to do is start fasting after dinner on one day, then continue the fast until dinnertime (at the same time) the following evening. Ideally, you will 'clean fast' during that period, but 'dirty fasting' is also fine (see page 57). Yes, you can have coffee with that. (No fries though, soz. Save those for tomorrow.)

**HOW OFTEN SHOULD I DO IT?**
Post-fast, you might feel so fab that you'll be tempted to do this regularly. While there is nothing wrong with a reset every now and again, trying to incorporate it as a regular part of your new life could be setting the fasting bar too high. Remember, the trick is to find what works for you long-term: 24-hour fast reset in moderation.

# Lana

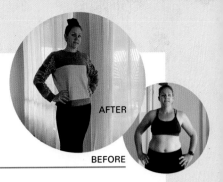

**LOST** 18 kg   Size 14 to size 10

**AFTER**

**BEFORE**

Eighteen months after having her twins, Lana just couldn't seem to shift the weight she'd gained. In fact, she kept gaining more. She tried everything, including exercising hard at the gym, but it wasn't until she tried SFD that the weight came off. When she plateaued, she used 24-hour fasts to blast her way forward. Back on track, she reached her goal, losing a life-changing 18 kg. 'After having my babies, I couldn't shift my weight and I was just getting bigger and bigger,' Lana says. 'I felt miserable, sad, ugly and fat. I was not even someone I recognised anymore, not only on the outside but on the inside as well.'

Lana went to the gym 3–4 times a week and tried everything, especially diet shakes, but it didn't work. 'I felt like a former shadow of myself, but a larger one and disgusting.' Then she found SFD. 'I was a bit sceptical at first as there was so much food to eat but that was the one main difference I could see between this program and all the others I tried: it wasn't restrictive. While hesitant, I gave it a go, and the weight just fell off. My favourite method is the part-day/16:8; I'm not a breakfast person and find it super easy to fast until lunchtime and miss that morning meal. It suits my lifestyle perfectly.'

Lana was losing weight steadily; however, she then hit a plateau. 'I had stalled in my weight loss for three weeks straight, so I learnt more about extended fasting and decided to try a 24-hour fast. I wasn't sure if it would be too hard but it's really just dinner to dinner – so doable once you're used to fasting for 16 hours. I know I can enjoy a nice dinner at the end of the day and most of the fasting hours are done while asleep so it makes it fairly easy to just do the one meal a day.

'This did it for me and I lost 1.1 kg that week. I then went on to lose double the amount of weight to 18 kg all up! Now I do 24-hour fasts once every 2–3 months as I find that's the most beneficial for my body. Doing them too often, I find I don't get the impact that I'm wanting from it so I try to use them for that power boost and it works great!

'I have so much energy now and am loving being fit, toned and healthy, and being active again daily,' Lana says. 'This program works. Who would have thought you can diet part-time, eat plenty of food and drop the kilos? Best way of life ever.'

**'Now I do 24-hour fasts once every 2-3 months as I find that's the most beneficial for my body ... I use them for that power boost and it works great!'**

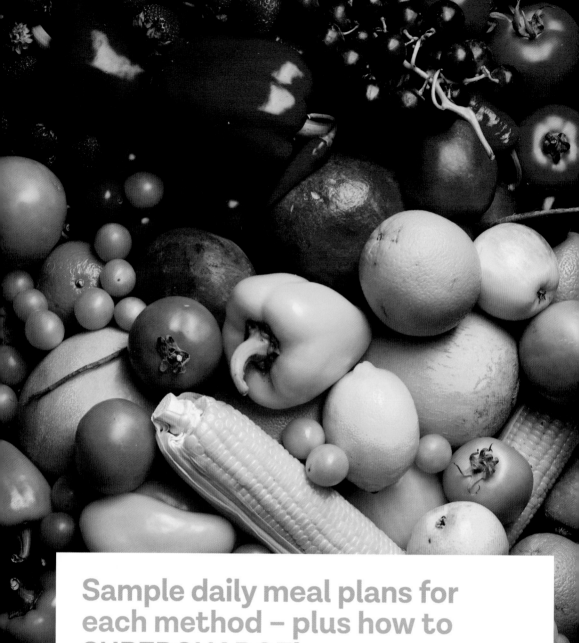

# Sample daily meal plans for each method – plus how to SUPERCHARGE!

At Superfastdiet.com we teach you how to plan your own meals so you can eat and drink pretty much ANYTHING in moderation and still lose weight! It's super flexible! However, on the following pages we have created some sample meal plans for you to follow until you get the hang of preparing your own. Feel free to swap anything out for a food/drink with a similar calorie count. The recipes starting on page 116 are also all calorie counted and nutritionally balanced for you, making The Fastest Diet also the easiest and yummiest diet on the planet!

# 2-day method

On the 2-day method, you choose two days a week to consume no more than 500 calories (600 calories for men), and on the other five days you can consume up to 2000 calories (2400 calories for men). Note: These calorie amounts are based on the average person. To calculate your exact calories see page 59. The 2-day method is a great way to get your fast days over and done with, then you can eat pretty much normally the rest of the week. Here are our top three tips for making the 2-day method work for you.

1 Choose your two fasting days for when you know you'll be busy, then have an early night.

2 Keep up the positive self-talk – mindset is everything!

3 Start with our sample meal plan to make it super easy and simple.

| | Sample 2-day method (500 cals) |
|---|---|
| **On rising** | Start the day with a lemon water<br>Herbal/fruit tea or tea/coffee with a splash of milk (10 cals) |
| **Breakfast** | 1 serve of Apple Pie & Creamy Yoghurt Bowl (194 cals) (see page 126)<br>OR 1 slice of toast with ½ banana |
| **Lunch** | 1 serve of Cucumber Cream Cheese Sandwiches (93 cals) (see page 208)<br>OR large green salad + 1 x 95 g can tuna in springwater + dash of balsamic vinegar |
| **Dinner** | 100 g choice of grilled lean turkey breast, white fish or pork fillet + your choice of spice mix and pepper for seasoning + 1 cup steamed broccolini and/or green beans – use olive oil spray, no butter (185 cals) |
| **Snacks** | ½ punnet strawberries (40 cals) |
| **Evening** | Herbal tea |
| **Drinks** | 2.5 litres water – still and/or sparkling (can infuse with fresh fruit, e.g. lemon, lime, orange)<br>Cup of tea/coffee with a splash of almond milk (3 cals)<br>Unlimited black tea and coffee<br>1 zero sugar soda, e.g. Coke No Sugar (not good for you but feel free if it gets you through the day)<br>Diet cordial – preferably naturally sweetened (6 cals)<br>250 ml (1 cup)/1 small bottle kombucha (30 cals) |

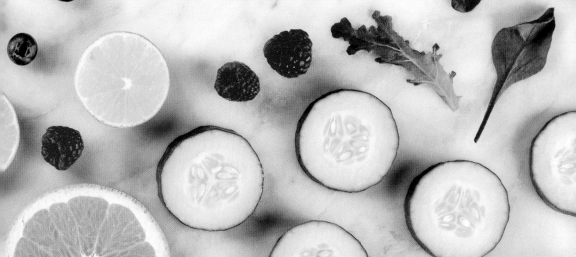

# 3-day method

On the 3-day method, you choose three days a week to consume no more than 1000 calories (1200 calories for men), and on the other four days you can consume up to 2000 calories (2400 calories for men). Note: These calorie amounts are based on the average person. To calculate your exact calories see page 59. The 3-day method can be an easier way for people to start with intermittent fasting as 1000 calories can go a long way. Here are our top three tips for making the 3-day method work for you.

1 Choose your three fasting days either all in a row or spaced out over the week to suit your lifestyle.

2 Fill up on black tea/fruit teas/coffee (you can add a splash of milk) and broth between meals and drink plenty of water.

3 Start with our meal plan to make it super easy and simple.

| | Sample 3-day method (1000 cals) |
|---|---|
| On rising | Start the day with a lemon water<br>Herbal/fruit tea or tea/coffee with a splash of milk (10 cals) |
| Breakfast | 1 serve of Caramel Chai Overnight Oats (212 cals) (see page 120)<br>OR 1 poached egg on a slice of wholemeal toast + 10 cherry tomatoes + a handful of English spinach |
| Lunch | 2 x 25 g mountain bread wraps + 50 g protein of choice (chicken, ham, tinned tuna) + ¾ cup mixed leafy green salad leaves and vegetables (lettuce, spinach, tomatoes, cucumber, carrot, capsicum) – divide the protein, salad greens and veg between the wraps (264 cals) |
| Dinner | 1 serve of Chargrilled Sumac Chicken with Not-So-Fattoush Salad (389 cals) (see page 174) |
| Snacks | 1 thick rice cake + ½ tbsp almond/peanut butter (85 cals)<br>OR 2 cups chopped watermelon |
| Evening | Herbal tea |
| Drinks | 2.5 litres water – still and/or sparkling (can infuse with fresh fruit, e.g. lemon, lime, orange)<br>Cup of tea/coffee with a splash of almond milk (3 cals)<br>Unlimited black tea and coffee<br>1 zero-sugar soda, e.g. Coke No Sugar (not good for you but feel free if it gets you through the day)<br>Diet cordial – preferably naturally sweetened (6 cals)<br>250 ml (1 cup)/1 small bottle kombucha (30 cals) |

# Part-day method

On the part-day method, you consume all of your calories for the day in an eight-hour window and fast for the other 16 hours a day. The calorie allowance is 1600 calories (2000 calories for men). Note: These calorie amounts are based on the average person. To calculate your exact calories see page 59. The part-day method can be as simple as skipping breakfast and, in an eight-hour eating window, 1600 calories is potentially a lot of food. Here are our top three tips for making the part-day method work for you.

**1** Choose what eight-hour eating hours will suit your lifestyle, e.g. most people like 12 pm –8 pm.

**2** If you're skipping breakfast, fill up on black teas, fruit teas or coffee instead (you can even have an almond milk cappuccino as you can have up to around 50 calories in your fasting window).

**3** Start with our meal plan to make it super easy and simple.

| | Sample part-day method (1600 cals) |
|---|---|
| **On rising** | Start the day with a lemon water<br>Herbal/fruit tea or tea/coffee with a splash of milk (**10 cals**) |
| **Mid-morning** | Cup of tea with a splash of almond milk (**3 cals**) |
| **Brunch at 11am–noon** | 1 serve of Herby Olive Frittata To Go (**292 cals**) (see page 142) |
| **Late snack** | 1 small slice (38 g) sourdough or wholegrain toast + 1 tbsp peanut butter + 1 small banana, sliced + 1 tsp chia seed sprinkled on top (**300 cals**) |
| **Dinner** | 1 serve of Smoky Shredded Pork Tacos (**405 cals**) (see page 184) |
| **Additional snacks** | 1 regular cappuccino with milk of choice (**101 cals**)<br>1 cup air-popped popcorn (**31 cals**)<br>1 serve of Chocolate Crackle Bites (**101 cals**) recipe on page 214<br>10 raw almonds (**70 cals**)<br>1 small banana (**77 cals**)<br>2 mango cheeks (**132 cals**) |
| **Evening** | Herbal tea |
| **Drinks** | 2.5 litres water – still and/or sparkling (can infuse with fresh fruit, e.g. lemon, lime, orange)<br>Cup of tea/coffee with a splash of almond milk (**3 cals**)<br>Unlimited black tea and coffee<br>1 zero-sugar soda, e.g. Coke No Sugar (not good for you but feel free if it gets you through the day)<br>Diet cordial – preferably naturally sweetened (**6 cals**)<br>250 ml (1 cup)/1 small bottle kombucha (**30 cals**) |

# Now for the magic of The Fastest Diet – let's SUPERCHARGE!

Welcome to supercharged weight-loss transformation! These sample meal plans unveil the extraordinary power of combining intermittent fasting methods, propelling you towards accelerated fat burn, increased energy and unrivalled results. Experience the transformative magic that lies within the fusion of intermittent fasting methods.

To supercharge, simply combine 2-day or 3-day with part-day – i.e. either eat all your 500 (600 for men) fasting-day calorie allowance in an eight-hour window (2-day combo) or eat all your 1000 (1200 for men) fasting day calorie allowance in an eight-hour window (3-day combo). Then for the rest of the week try to continue eating in your eight-hour window i.e. follow the part-day method plan.

**FINISH EATING WINDOW BY 7 OR 8 PM, DEPENDING ON WHEN YOU COMMENCED EATING.**

| | Sample 2-day method combo (500 cals in an eight-hour window) |
|---|---|
| **On rising** | Start the day with a lemon water<br>Herbal/fruit tea or tea/coffee with a splash of milk (**10 cals**) |
| **Mid-morning** | Cup of tea/coffee with a splash of almond milk (**3 cals**) |
| **Brunch at 11am–noon** | 1 serve of Chilli Peanut Fried Eggs (**187 cals**) (see page 122)<br>OR 1 poached egg + slice of wholemeal toast + a side of English spinach |
| **Dinner** | 1 serve of 3-Minute Red Curry Noodles (**290 cals**) (see page 146) |
| **Snacks** | Cup of tea with a splash of almond milk (**3 cals**)<br>½ cup cucumber and celery sticks (**16 cals**) |
| **Evening** | Herbal tea |
| **Drinks** | 2.5 litres water – still and/or sparkling (can infuse with fresh fruit, e.g. lemon, lime, orange)<br>Cup of tea/coffee with a splash of almond milk (**3 cals**)<br>Unlimited black tea and coffee<br>1 zero-sugar soda, e.g. Coke No Sugar (not good for you but feel free if it gets you through the day)<br>Diet cordial – preferably naturally sweetened (**6 cals**)<br>250 ml (1 cup)/1 small bottle kombucha (**30 cals**) |

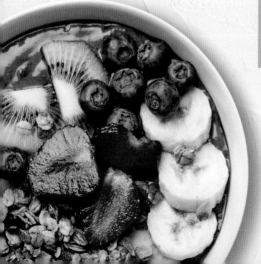

| | Sample 3-day method combo (1000 cals in an eight-hour window) |
|---|---|
| On rising | Start the day with a lemon water<br>Herbal/fruit tea or tea/coffee with a splash of milk (10 cals) |
| Mid-morning | Cup of tea/coffee with a splash of almond milk (3 cals) |
| Brunch at 11am–noon | 1 serve of Reuben Club Sandwich (310 cals) (see page 158)<br>OR fresh green salad with your fave chopped raw veggies such as cherry tomatoes, cucumber, radish, sliced carrots, red onion, mushrooms, capsicum with 14 almonds + a squeeze of lemon juice and a dash of balsamic vinegar + 100 g cooked chicken or lean protein of your choice |
| Dinner | 1 serve of Fish with Blistering Tomatoes Tray Bake (391 cals) (see page 189) |
| Snacks | 1 serve of Salt & Vinegar Edamame (100 cals) (see page 210)<br>250 ml (1 cup) instant miso soup (35 cals)<br>40 g (¼ cup) blueberries (21 cals)<br>1 kiwifruit (40 cals)<br>Cup of tea with a splash of almond milk (3 cals)<br>1 regular cappuccino with milk of choice (101 cals) |
| Evening | Herbal tea |
| Drinks | 2.5 litres water – still and/or sparkling (can infuse with fresh fruit, e.g. lemon, lime, orange)<br>Cup of tea/coffee with a splash of almond milk (3 cals)<br>Unlimited black tea and coffee<br>1 zero-sugar soda, e.g. Coke No Sugar (not good for you but feel free if it gets you through the day)<br>Diet cordial – preferably naturally sweetened (6 cals)<br>250 ml (1 cup)/1 small bottle kombucha (30 cals) |

# Supercharge sample weekly meal plan

For those of you who are really new to fasting, including a whole week's plan is probably going to be super helpful. Here you will find a seven-day meal plan that combines our 3-day method with the time-restricted principles of our part-day method. Note that on three of the seven days your calories are set at 1000 calories per day and the other four days are set at 1600 calories, which is taken from our part-day method. We call this supercharging. Read more on page 28.

Note: You can combine the calories from brunch and late snack to be one meal at lunchtime, if you prefer.

**FINISH EATING WINDOW BY 7 OR 8 PM, DEPENDING ON WHEN YOU COMMENCED EATING.**

| | Day 1 (3-day/1000 cals) |
|---|---|
| **On rising** | Start the day with a lemon water<br>Herbal/fruit tea or tea/coffee with a splash of milk (**10 cals**) |
| **Mid-morning** | Cup of tea with a splash of almond milk (**3 cals**) |
| **Brunch at 11 am–noon** | 1 serve of Miracle Bagels (**298 cals**) (see page 140) |
| **Late snack** | 1 small slice (38 g) sourdough or wholegrain toast + ¼ smashed avocado + 30 g (½ cup) rocket + 2 medium sliced tomatoes + freshly ground black pepper (**178 cals**) |
| **Dinner** | 1 serve of BBQ Chicken Steaks with Chargrilled Vegetables (**391 cals**) (see page 166) |
| **Additional snacks** | 1 regular cappuccino with milk of choice (**101 cals**)<br>40 g (¼ cup) fresh blueberries (**21 cals**)<br>¼ punnet strawberries (**20 cals**)<br>Cup of tea with a splash of almond milk (**3 cals**) |
| **Evening** | Herbal tea |
| **Drinks** | 2.5 litres water – still and/or sparkling (can infuse with fresh fruit, e.g. lemon, lime, orange)<br>Cup of tea/coffee with a splash of almond milk (**3 cals**)<br>Unlimited black tea and coffee<br>1 zero-sugar soda, e.g. Coke No Sugar (not good for you but feel free if it gets you through the day)<br>Diet cordial – preferably naturally sweetened (**6 cals**)<br>250 ml (1 cup)/1 small bottle kombucha (**30 cals**) |

| Day 2 (part-day/1600 cals) | Day 3 (3-day/1000 cals) |
|---|---|
| Start the day with a lemon water<br>Herbal/fruit tea or tea/coffee with a splash of milk (10 cals) | Start the day with a lemon water<br>Herbal/fruit tea or tea/coffee with a splash of milk (10 cals) |
| Cup of tea with a splash of almond milk (3 cals) | Cup of tea with a splash of almond milk (3 cals) |
| 1 serve of Smoky Chickpea & Capsicum Scramble (297 cals) (see page 134) | 1 serve of Peanut Tuna Wrap with Torn Leaves & Fennel (303 cals) (see page 152) |
| 120 g yoghurt (dairy, coconut, almond) + 40 g (¼ cup) fresh or frozen blueberries + 1 small sliced banana + ½ tbsp honey + 10 g flaked almonds (342 cals) | 1 serve of Raspberry Rose Smoothie (97 cals) (see page 128) |
| 1 serve of Resting Roast Chicken on Ratatouille Bed + 1 slice (50 g) toasted crusty sourdough (581 cals) (see page 168) | 120 g lean protein (beef, pork fillet, chicken or fish) + 2 cups steamed broccolini and/or green beans + ½ cup steamed/mashed/dry roasted sweet potato<br>Only use olive oil spray, no butter. Season protein with your choice of spice mix and pepper and cook as desired. (369 cals) |
| 1 regular cappuccino with milk of choice (101 cals)<br>3 small watermelon wedges (63 cals)<br>1 cup air-popped popcorn (31 cals)<br>3 squares of Lindt 70 per cent dark chocolate (170 cals) | 1 regular cappuccino with milk of choice (101 cals)<br>⅓ cup edamame beans (62 cals)<br>1 kiwi fruit (40 cals)<br>1 cup air-popped popcorn (31 cals)<br>Cup of tea with a splash of almond milk (3 cals) |
| Herbal tea | Herbal tea |
| 2.5 litres water – still and/or sparkling (can infuse with fresh fruit, e.g. lemon, lime, orange)<br>Cup of tea/coffee with a splash of almond milk (3 cals)<br>Unlimited black tea and coffee<br>1 zero-sugar soda, e.g. Coke No Sugar (not good for you but feel free if it gets you through the day)<br>Diet cordial – preferably naturally sweetened (6 cals)<br>250 ml (1 cup)/1 small bottle kombucha (30 cals) | 2.5 litres water – still and/or sparkling (can infuse with fresh fruit, e.g. lemon, lime, orange)<br>Cup of tea/coffee with a splash of almond milk (3 cals)<br>Unlimited black tea and coffee<br>1 zero-sugar soda, e.g. Coke No Sugar (not good for you but feel free if it gets you through the day)<br>Diet cordial – preferably naturally sweetened (6 cals)<br>250 ml (1 cup)/1 small bottle kombucha (30 cals) |

| | Day 4 (part-day/1600 cals) | Day 5 (3-day/1000 cals) |
|---|---|---|
| **On rising** | Start the day with a lemon water<br><br>Herbal/fruit tea or tea/coffee with a splash of milk (**10 cals**) | Start the day with a lemon water<br><br>Herbal/fruit tea or tea/coffee with a splash of milk (**10 cals**) |
| **Mid-morning** | Cup of tea with a splash of almond milk (**3 cals**) | Cup of tea with a splash of almond milk (**3 cals**) |
| **Brunch at 11 am–noon** | 1 serve of Curry Tofu & Cauliflower Tray Bake (**399 cals**) (see page 198) | 1 serve of Green Goddess Egg Salad Open Sandwich (**300 cals**) (see page 151) |
| **Late snack** | 1 small slice (38 g) of sourdough or wholegrain toast + 1 tbsp peanut butter + 1 small sliced banana, sliced + 1 tsp chia seeds, sprinkled on top (**293 cals**) | 1 small watermelon wedge, chopped + 40 g (¼ cup) fresh blueberries + 1 kiwi fruit, chopped + 1 scoop passionfruit pulp + 10 g flaked almonds (**161 cals**) |
| **Dinner** | 1 serve of BBQ Steak Fajita Bowl + 2 x 25 g mini tortillas (**549 cals**) (see page 180) | 1 serve of Love This Jerk Salmon with Marinated Tomato Salsa (**401 cals**) (see page 192) |
| **Additional snacks** | 1 regular cappuccino with milk of choice (**101 cals**)<br><br>1 serve of Oaty Peach Crumble (**103 cals**) (see page 212)<br><br>1 x 40 g store-bought or homemade protein ball (**165 cals**)<br><br>¼ punnet strawberries (**20 cals**) | 1 regular cappuccino with milk of choice (**101 cals**)<br><br>1 cup air-popped popcorn (**31 cals**)<br><br>Cup of tea with a splash of almond milk (**3 cals**) |
| **Evening** | Herbal tea | Herbal tea |
| **Drinks** | 2.5 litres water – still and/or sparkling (can infuse with fresh fruit, e.g. lemon, lime, orange)<br><br>Cup of tea/coffee with a splash of almond milk (**3 cals**)<br><br>Unlimited black tea and coffee<br><br>1 zero-sugar soda, e.g. Coke No Sugar (not good for you but feel free if it gets you through the day)<br><br>Diet cordial – preferably naturally sweetened (**6 cals**)<br><br>250 ml (1 cup)/1 small bottle kombucha (**30 cals**) | 2.5 litres water – still and/or sparkling (can infuse with fresh fruit, e.g. lemon, lime, orange)<br><br>Cup of tea/coffee with a splash of almond milk (**3 cals**)<br><br>Unlimited black tea and coffee<br><br>1 zero-sugar soda, e.g. Coke No Sugar (not good for you but feel free if it gets you through the day)<br><br>Diet cordial – preferably naturally sweetened (**6 cals**)<br><br>250 ml (1 cup)/1 small bottle kombucha (**30 cals**) |

| Day 6 (part-day/1600 cals) | Day 7 (part-day/1600 cals) |
|---|---|
| Start the day with a lemon water<br>Herbal/fruit tea or tea/coffee with a splash of milk (10 cals) | Start the day with a lemon water<br>Herbal/fruit tea or tea/coffee with a splash of milk (10 cals) |
| Cup of tea with a splash of almond milk (3 cals) | Cup of tea with a splash of almond milk (3 cals) |
| 1 serve of Chilli Prawn Omelette + 100 g (½ cup) brown or jasmine rice (522 cals) (see page 190) | 1 serve of Ultimate Chicken Power Bowls + ¼ cup cooked quinoa + 1 tbsp dry-roasted pumpkin seeds (420 cals) (see page 154)<br>Or brekkie out earlier... |
| 2 x 40 g store-bought or homemade protein balls (330 cals) | 2 serves of Cucumber Cream Cheese Sandwiches (194 cals) (see page 208) |
| 1 serve of Chargrilled Green Tomatoes & Lamb Chops with Pickled Yoghurt + ½ cup steamed/mashed/dry roasted sweet potato (550 cals) (see page 182) | 1 serve of Tomato & Fish-in-a-Curry + 95 g (½ cup) basmati rice (500 cals) (see page 188) |
| 1 regular cappuccino with milk of choice (101 cals)<br>1 cup green grapes (100 cals) | 1 regular cappuccino with milk of choice (101 cals)<br>180 g (1 cup) green grapes (100 cals)<br>1 small banana (77 cals)<br>3 squares of Lindt 70 per cent dark chocolate (170 cals) |
| Herbal tea | Herbal tea |
| 2.5 litres water – still and/or sparkling (can infuse with fresh fruit, e.g. lemon, lime, orange)<br>Cup of tea/coffee with a splash of almond milk (3 cals)<br>Unlimited black tea and coffee<br>1 zero-sugar soda, e.g. Coke No Sugar (not good for you but feel free if it gets you through the day)<br>Diet cordial – preferably naturally sweetened (6 cals)<br>250 ml (1 cup)/1 small bottle kombucha (30 cals) | 2.5 litres water – still and/or sparkling (can infuse with fresh fruit, e.g. lemon, lime, orange)<br>Cup of tea/coffee with a splash of almond milk (3 cals)<br>Unlimited black tea and coffee<br>1 zero-sugar soda, e.g. Coke No Sugar (not good for you but feel free if it gets you through the day)<br>Diet cordial – preferably naturally sweetened (6 cals)<br>250 ml (1 cup)/1 small bottle kombucha (30 cals) |

On this day you can choose to stick to the plan or if you prefer, why not take a day off time restricted eating and enjoy 'brekkie' out at your favourite cafe! Easiest way to do this is skip our Ultimate Chicken Power Bowl brunch and instead you've got 420 calories up your sleeve to enjoy a delish breakfast treat. You'll easily fit two poached eggs on crusty sourdough toast with a side of smashed avocado plus a coffee into that calories allowance. Go on, you've earned it!

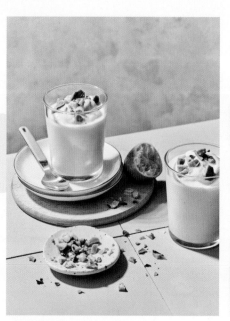
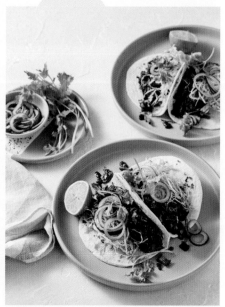
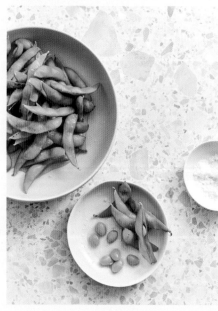
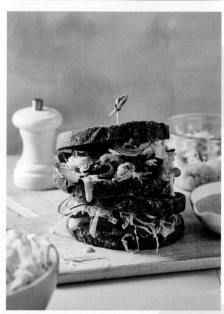

# Recipes

We have created these ultra-divine recipes for you to mix and match on both your fast days and non-fast days. They are all super low-calorie yet absolutely delicious, extraordinarily nutrient-dense AND easy to make!

To plan your day, simply choose a breakfast, brunch and/or lunch, add a main and then a snack or two! Make sure the total calories are under your daily target and you're ready to rock 'n' roll!

Although we have divided the recipes into traditional mealtimes, they can all be eaten at any time of the day to suit your chosen eating window. Feel free to have a lunch recipe for dinner or a breakfast recipe for lunch.

Please don't feel pressured to use a recipe for every meal – you can be totally flexible by adding in no-recipe meals – just make sure the ingredients you use are in line with your daily calorie allowance. See our sample meal plans for each method on page 107 for ideas.

Remember, we don't want you to be deprived! Add in some dark chocolate, cheese and crackers and a lovely glass of wine with dinner if desired. Whatever floats your boat.

'Everything in moderation ... including moderation.'

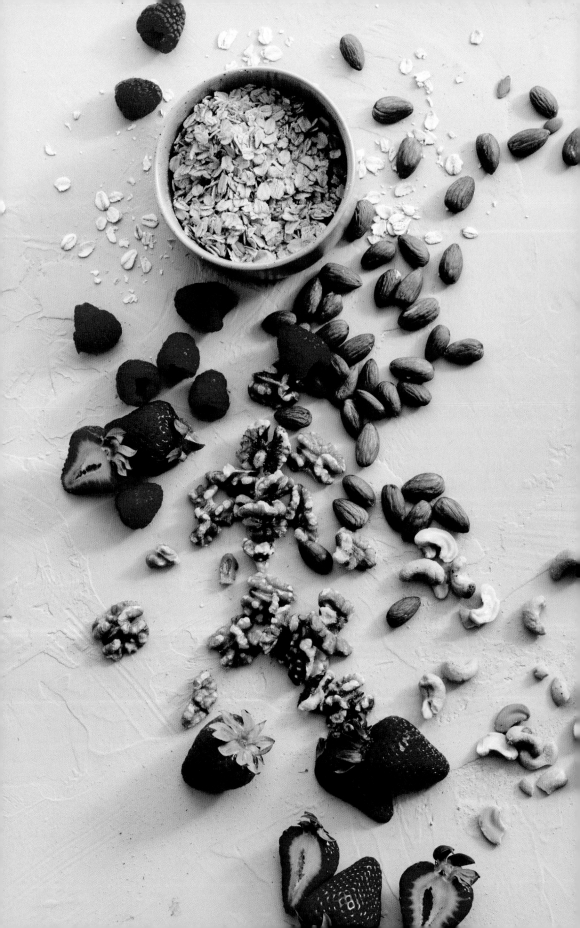

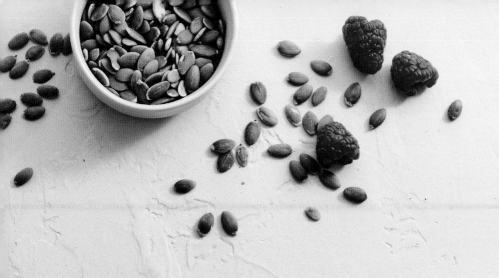

# Breakfast

Whether you're breakfasting in the morning or the middle of the day – or in fact any time you want to start your eating window – these totally scrummy and easy-to-make recipes will tantalise your taste buds and leave you feeling energised ... without the high calories.

So go ahead and indulge in some breakfast goodness at any time of the day! #breakfastwithsass

# Caramel Chai Overnight Oats

**Get two breakfasts in one with this warming chai tea and porridge duo, all wrapped into one nourishing, comforting breakfast.**

375 ml (1½ cups) unsweetened almond milk
2 chai tea bags
100 g (1 cup) rolled oats
1 teaspoon vanilla bean powder
500 ml (2 cups) water
2 teaspoons honey
1 tablespoon shredded coconut

Add the almond milk to a medium saucepan over medium heat and bring to the boil. Reduce the heat to low, add the chai tea bags and simmer for 3–4 minutes (depending how strong you'd like the chai flavour), then remove the tea bags. Add the oats and vanilla and cook, stirring, for about 5 minutes, adding as much of the water as needed to reach the consistency you like.

Divide the porridge between two bowls, top with the honey and coconut flakes and serve.

**Note** To prepare overnight, instead of cooking the oats, add them to a container and pour the warm chai milk over the top. Stir to combine, then place in the fridge for the oats to soak up the mixture overnight.

## BOOST

⌃ Serve with 1 tablespoon of low-fat natural yoghurt.
Extra 11 calories per serve.

**SERVES**
2

**PREP**
2 minutes

**COOK**
10 minutes

**CALS PER SERVE**
212

**DAIRY FREE**

**15 MINUTES OR LESS**

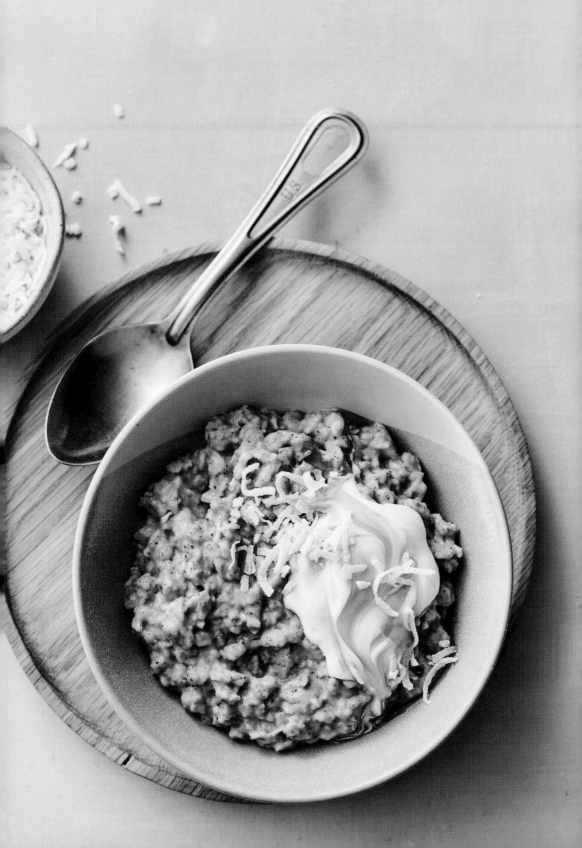

# Chilli Peanut Fried Eggs

With the addition of chilli, these sunny eggs will give you a bright kickstart to your day! Protein-rich and packed with peanutty crunch, you'll feel full and energised for hours.

1 teaspoon extra-virgin olive oil

4 free-range eggs

½–1 teaspoon chilli flakes

4 thin slices wholemeal bread, toasted

10 g butter

40 g (¼ cup) dry-roasted peanuts, roughly chopped

2 tablespoons finely chopped spring onion

150 g (1 cup) cherry tomatoes, halved

Sea salt flakes

Heat the oil in a large non-stick frying pan over medium–high heat. Once hot, crack the eggs into the pan and sprinkle the chilli flakes around the edges. Cook for 4–5 minutes, until the egg whites are set.

Butter the toast and divide between four plates. Top with the fried eggs, then sprinkle with the peanuts and spring onion. Serve with the cherry tomatoes and season the lot with the salt and some freshly ground black pepper.

---

### BOOST

⌃ Add 2 teaspoons of Homemade Labne (page 222) for a creamy and tangy addition to these fried eggs. Extra 25 calories per serve.

---

| SERVES | PREP | COOK | CALS PER SERVE | DAIRY FREE | VEGETARIAN | 15 MINUTES OR LESS |
|---|---|---|---|---|---|---|
| 4 | 5 minutes | 5 minutes | 187 | | | |

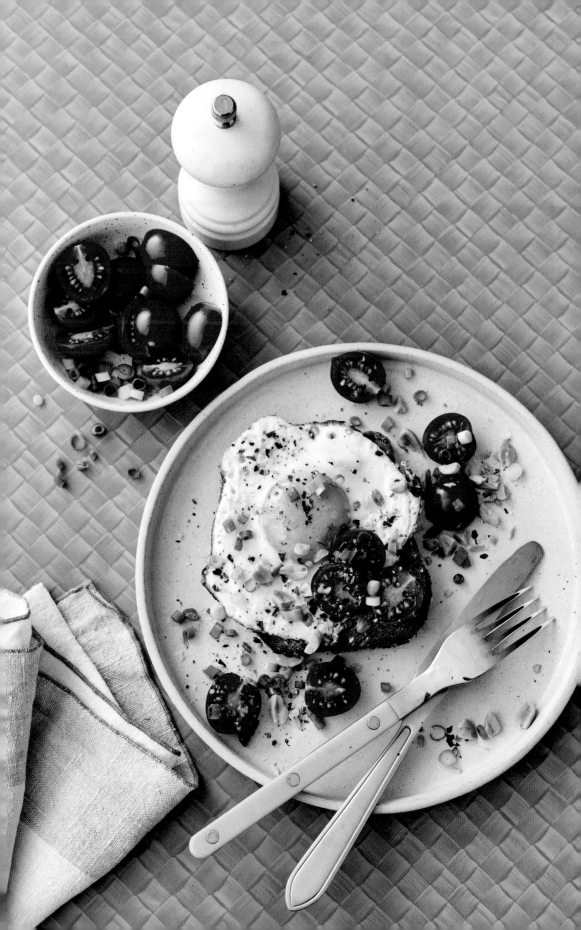

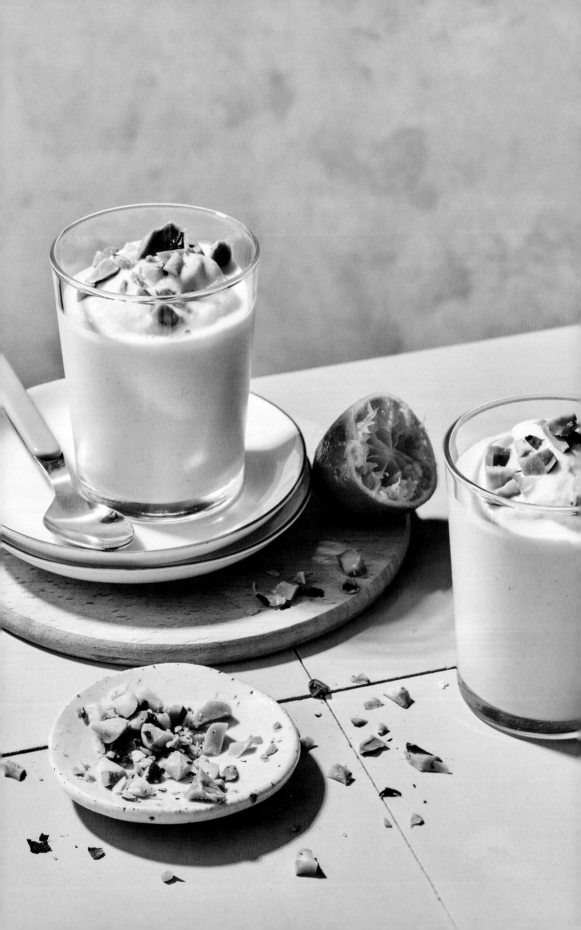

# Brazilian Mango Whip

Who says you can't have a cocktail for breakfast? And when it's packed full of tropical flavour and topped with buttery brazil nuts, you'd have to be troppo (or nuts) to say no!

150 g (1 cup) frozen mango

125 g (½ cup) low-fat natural yoghurt, frozen in an ice-cube tray

125 g (½ cup) low-fat natural yoghurt

2 tablespoons vanilla protein powder

Juice of 1 lime

125–185 ml (½–¾ cup) water

3 brazil nuts, finely chopped

Add the frozen mango, yoghurt ice cubes, yoghurt, protein powder and lime juice to a blender. Add a dash of the water and blitz on high until smooth. Add more water as needed to blend until smooth and thick.

Divide between two glasses and top with the chopped brazil nuts to serve.

## Note

» To prepare this smoothie ahead of time, freeze a whole tub of yoghurt into standard ice cube trays. Once frozen, pop them out and store in an airtight container or ziplock bag in the freezer, ready to use.

» Freeze the smoothie into popsicle moulds for an icy-pole breakfast!

**SERVES** 2

**PREP** 5 minutes

**CALS PER SERVE** 200

**GLUTEN FREE**

**5 MINUTES OR LESS**

# Apple Pie & Creamy Yoghurt Bowl

Cinnamon is the perfect health hack to start your day as it helps regulate blood glucose levels and dulls sugar cravings. It also tastes like heaven when mixed with apple, lemon, maple syrup and coconut ... all golden and waiting for you on a creamy bed of yoghurt, sprinkled with walnuts. Sigh.

2 teaspoons chopped walnuts
1 large red apple, cored
  and roughly chopped
  into 1 cm chunks
½ teaspoon ground cinnamon
Juice of ½ lemon
250 g (1 cup) low-fat natural
  yoghurt
1 tablespoon shredded coconut
2 teaspoons maple syrup

Place a medium saucepan over medium heat and add the walnuts. Cook, stirring, for 2–3 minutes, until the walnuts are golden brown. Tip into a bowl and set aside.

Add the apple, cinnamon, lemon juice and 60 ml (¼ cup) water to the saucepan over medium–low heat. Cook, stirring, for 10 minutes until the apples are tender but still retain their shape.

Divide the yoghurt between two bowls and top with the stewed apples, then the toasted walnuts and shredded coconut. Drizzle with the maple syrup and serve.

**SERVES**
2

**PREP**
5 minutes

**COOK**
10 minutes

**CALS PER
SERVE**
194

**GLUTEN
FREE**

**15
MINUTES
OR LESS**

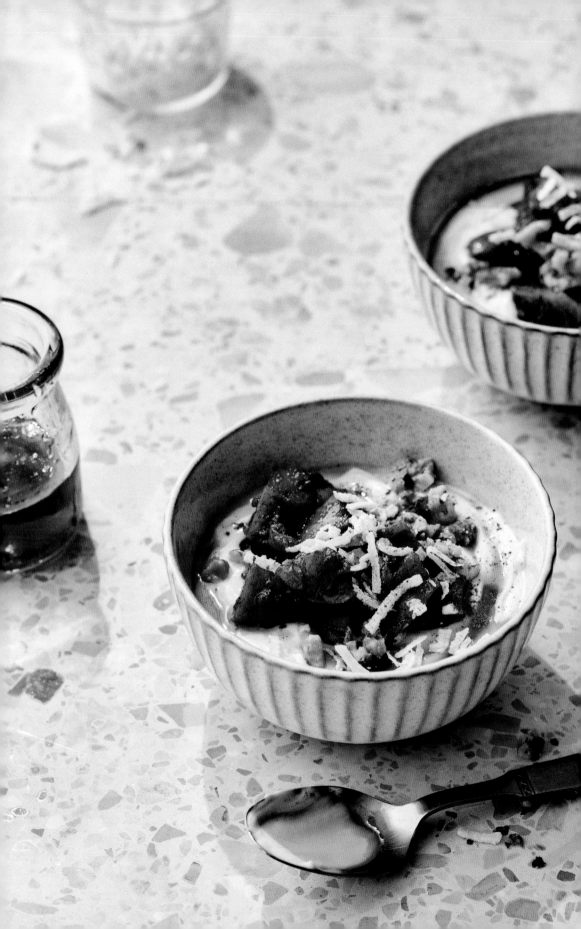

# Raspberry Rose Smoothie

Love at first sip! This rose-tinted vanilla and berry smoothie is a totally refreshing way to start your morning, or to have as an afternoon pick-me-up.

140 g (¾ cup) frozen raspberries

1 teaspoon natural vanilla extract

½ teaspoon rosewater

1 teaspoon chia seeds

60 ml (¼ cup) coconut milk, frozen into ice cubes

2 teaspoons honey

375 ml (1½ cups) unsweetened almond milk

Add all the ingredients to a blender and blitz on high until smooth. Divide between two glasses to serve.

**Note** To prepare the smoothie ahead of time, pour a 400 ml can of coconut milk into standard ice cube trays, then freeze. Once frozen, pop them out and store in an airtight container or ziplock bag in the freezer, ready to use.

---

**BOOST**

» Add 30 g (4 tablespoons) vanilla protein powder.
Extra 62 calories per serve.

---

**SERVES**
2

**PREP**
2 minutes,
plus freezing

**CALS PER SERVE**
97

**GLUTEN FREE**

**5 MINUTES OR LESS**

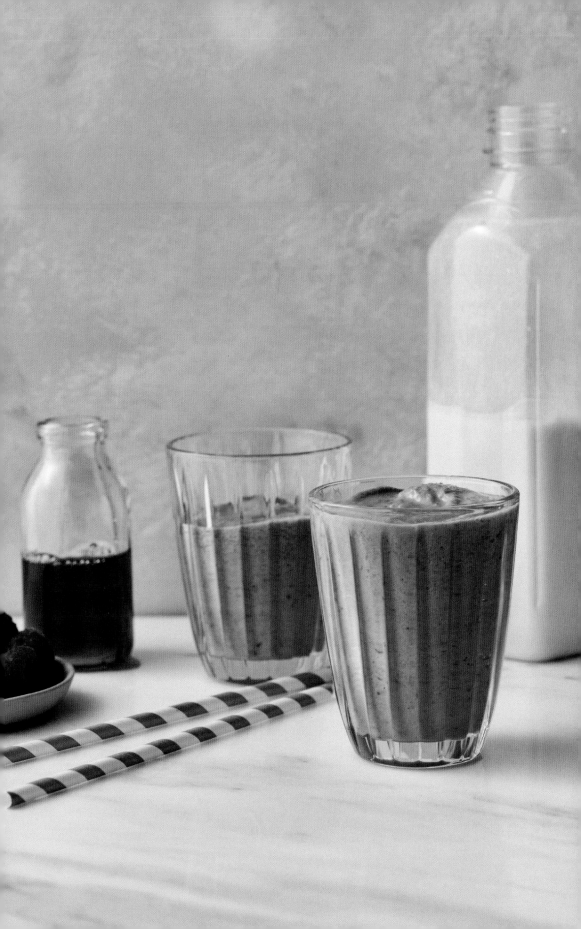

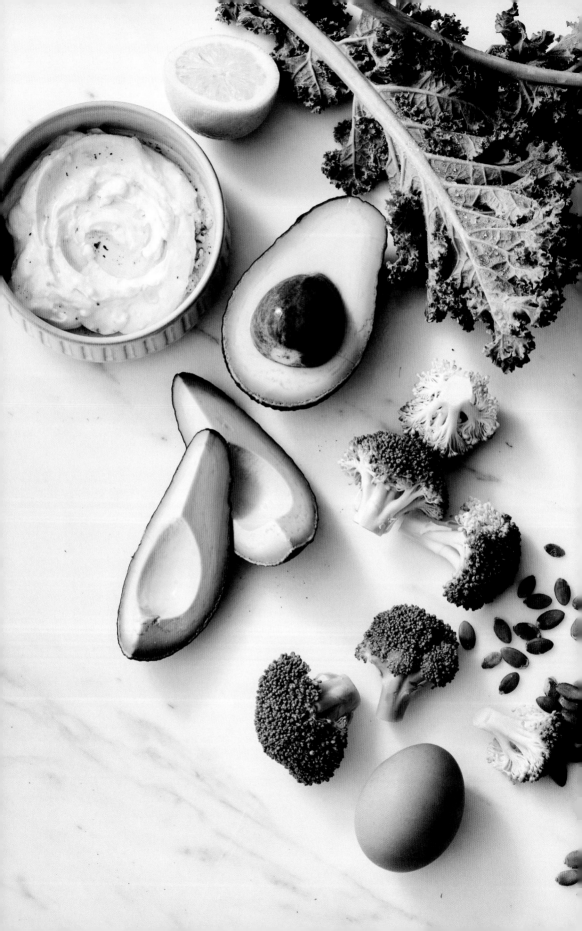

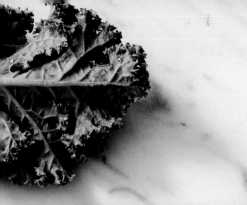

# Brunch

What do you get when you skip breakfast and combine it with lunch? A part-day fast – or Supercharging, if you're doing a combo with 2-day or 3-day.

'Brunch' is our fave meal-word here at SFD and you only have to look at these recipes to see why. From sweet to savoury, brunch recipes offer you a range of options, such as bagels, eggs, salads and frittatas.

Bonus brunch points! By the time you start your eating window you have worked up a healthy hunger and your food tastes AH-MAZING!

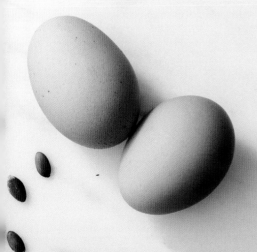

# White Bean Antipasto Salad

Fresh, delicious and vibrant in colour, how good does this dish look?
Perfect for brunch, this salad can be made in advance and left to marinate
overnight for the best flavour infusion.

2 x 400 g cans white beans,
 drained and rinsed
 (yields 3 cups of beans)
500 g cherry tomatoes,
 quartered
250 g artichoke hearts in brine,
 drained, rinsed and
 roughly chopped
2 bunches of asparagus, woody
 ends trimmed and spears
 chopped into 1 cm pieces
½ red onion, finely sliced
2 slices wholemeal or gluten-
 free bread, toasted and sliced
 in half into triangles

### DRESSING
Juice of 1 lemon
2 teaspoons extra-virgin olive oil
1 tablespoon capers in vinegar,
 finely chopped
¼ cup finely chopped flat-leaf
 parsley
½ teaspoon sea salt flakes
¼ teaspoon freshly ground
 black pepper

Add all the dressing ingredients to a jar and shake
to combine.

Add the white beans, cherry tomatoes, artichoke, asparagus
and red onion to a large bowl. Drizzle with the dressing and
toss gently to combine.

Divide the salad between four bowls and serve each with
half a slice of toast.

## BOOST

≫ Add 2 tablespoons of
 mayonnaise to the
 dressing. Extra 30 calories
 per serve.

|  SERVES 4 |  PREP 10 minutes |  COOK 3 minutes |  CALS PER SERVE 302 |  GLUTEN FREE |  DAIRY FREE |  VEGAN |  15 MINUTES OR LESS |

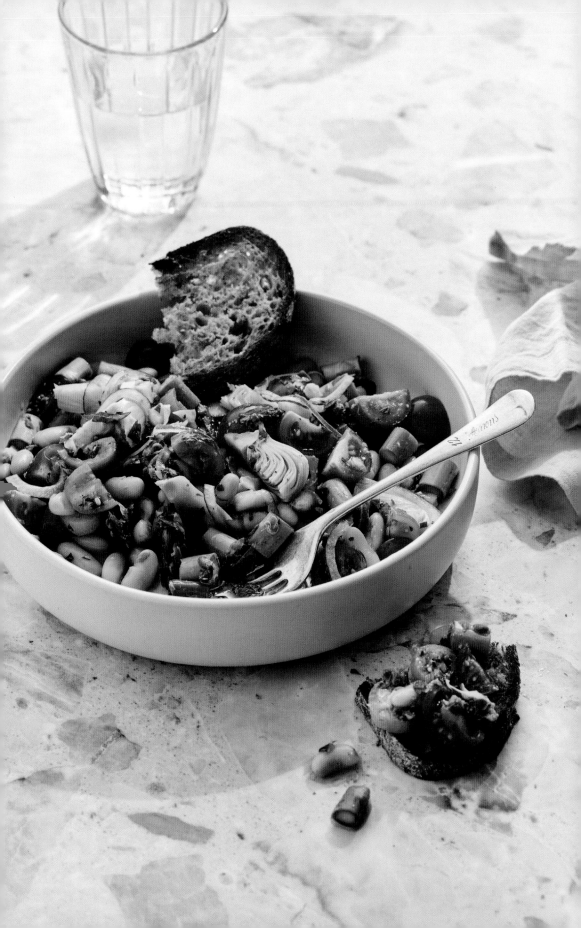

# Smoky Chickpea & Capsicum Scramble

They'll be scrambling to the table to enjoy this spicy, nourishing dish, with paprika and chilli adding deeply warming flavours that elevate this brunch to gourmet level!

4 free-range eggs

1 teaspoon extra-virgin olive oil

2 x 440 g cans chickpeas, drained and rinsed (yields 3 cups chickpeas)

3 red capsicums, deseeded and finely sliced

3 garlic cloves, minced

2 teaspoons smoked paprika (see notes)

1 teaspoon ground coriander

¼ teaspoon chilli powder

1 tablespoon chopped chives

Fill a medium saucepan with water and place over high heat. Once boiling, add the eggs and cook, undisturbed, for 6 minutes for soft-boiled egg, or 8 minutes for hard-boiled. Remove the eggs with a slotted spoon and run them under cool water until cool to the touch. Peel and cut in half.

While the eggs are cooking, heat the olive oil in a large frying pan over medium heat. Once hot, add the chickpeas and capsicum. Cook, tossing, for 1 minute, then add 2 tablespoons of water and place the lid on the frying pan. Continue to cook for 3 minutes, allowing the capsicum to steam until tender. Remove the lid and add the garlic, paprika, coriander and chilli powder. Cook, tossing, for 1 minute, until fragrant.

Divide the scramble between four bowls, topping each serve with a boiled egg and some chives.

## Notes

» Instead of the smoked paprika, ground coriander and chilli powder, you can substitute 3¼ teaspoons of store-bought Mexican spice blend.

» For brunches during the week, store individual portions in airtight containers. Reheat in the microwave for 1 minute on High until warmed through.

*BOOST*

☆ Serve with 1 tablespoon of low-fat natural yoghurt.
Extra 11 calories per serve.

| SERVES | PREP | COOK | CALS PER SERVE | GLUTEN FREE | DAIRY FREE | VEGETARIAN | 30 MINUTES OR LESS |
|---|---|---|---|---|---|---|---|
| 4 | 5 minutes | 15 minutes | 297 | | | | |

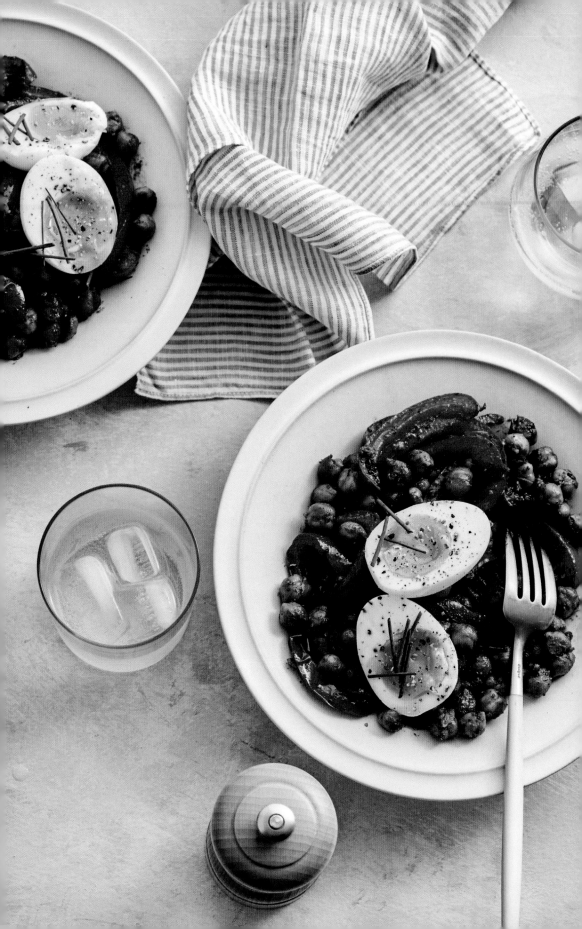

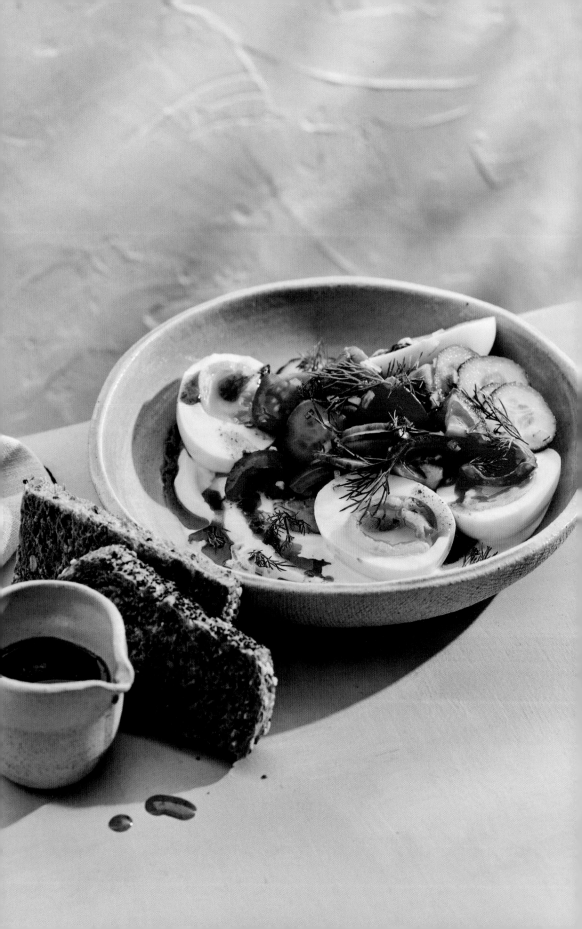

# Turkish Spiced Eggs

Dine cafe-style at home with this totally gooey, drizzly, exotically spiced dish. Simply boil the eggs for 6 minutes for the perfect brunch plate.

8 free-range eggs

2 tomatoes, diced

1 Lebanese cucumber,
   finely sliced

½ small red onion, finely diced

250 g (1 cup) low-fat natural
   yoghurt

1 tablespoon dill leaves

4 slices wholemeal bread,
   toasted, sliced in half

CHILLI OIL

1½ tablespoons extra-virgin
   olive oil

1 teaspoon cumin seeds

1 teaspoon smoked paprika

½ teaspoon chilli flakes

Fill a medium saucepan with water and place over high heat. Once boiling, add the eggs and cook, undisturbed, for 6 minutes. Remove the eggs with a slotted spoon and run them under cool water until cool to the touch. Peel and cut in half.

To make the chilli oil, heat the oil in a small non-stick frying pan over medium heat. Add the cumin seeds, paprika and chilli flakes and toast for 1 minute, until fragrant. Set aside.

Add the tomato, cucumber and onion to a bowl and toss to combine.

To serve, spread the yoghurt on the bottom of four small shallow bowls, then divide the eggs between the bowls. Top with the tomato salad and drizzle with the chilli oil. Garnish with the dill leaves and season with ¼ teaspoon freshly ground black pepper. Serve with wholemeal toast.

**SERVES**
4

**PREP**
5 minutes

**COOK**
15 minutes

**CALS PER SERVE**
309

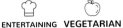
ENTERTAINING **VEGETARIAN**

**30 MINUTES OR LESS**

# The Bondi Brunch Salad

This salad is so hip and happening it almost looks too good to eat!
A wellness bowl overflowing with goodness, this salad is full of greens,
good fats and protein, with a beach cafe vibe that will leave you feeling
as fresh and fabulous as an ocean breeze.

4 free-range eggs

40 g (¼ cup) pumpkin seeds

1 head broccoli

4 cups shredded kale leaves

Juice of 1 lemon

2 teaspoons extra-virgin olive oil

½ teaspoon sea salt flakes

¼ cup chopped dill leaves

¼ cup chopped flat-leaf parsley

1 avocado, diced

75 g (⅓ cup) Homemade Labne
    (page 222)

Fill a medium saucepan with water and place over high heat. Once boiling, add the eggs and cook, undisturbed, for 6 minutes for soft-boiled, or 8 minutes for hard-boiled. Remove the eggs with a slotted spoon and run them under cool water until cool to the touch. Peel and cut in half. Set aside.

Heat a medium frying pan over medium–high heat. Add the pumpkin seeds and cook, tossing, for 3–5 minutes, until golden brown. Set aside.

Finely shred the broccoli, including the stem. You can do this with a sharp knife, grate it on a box grater, or blitz in a food processor. Add the broccoli to a large bowl with the shredded kale. Squeeze the lemon juice over the top, drizzle with the olive oil and season with the sea salt flakes and a pinch of freshly ground black pepper. Use your hands to toss the lemon through the greens, massaging and squeezing to tenderise them. Add the dill, parsley and avocado and toss them through.

Spread the labne on four serving plates. Top with the green salad and a boiled egg. Sprinkle with the toasted pumpkin seeds and serve.

This salad will keep for up to 5 days in the fridge.

---

**BOOST**

⌃ Serve with 2 teaspoons of tahini as a creamy nutty dressing. Extra 45 calories per serve.

---

| SERVES | PREP | COOK | CALS PER SERVE | GLUTEN FREE | VEGETARIAN | 30 MINUTES OR LESS |
|---|---|---|---|---|---|---|
| 4 | 10 minutes | 15 minutes | 297 | | | |

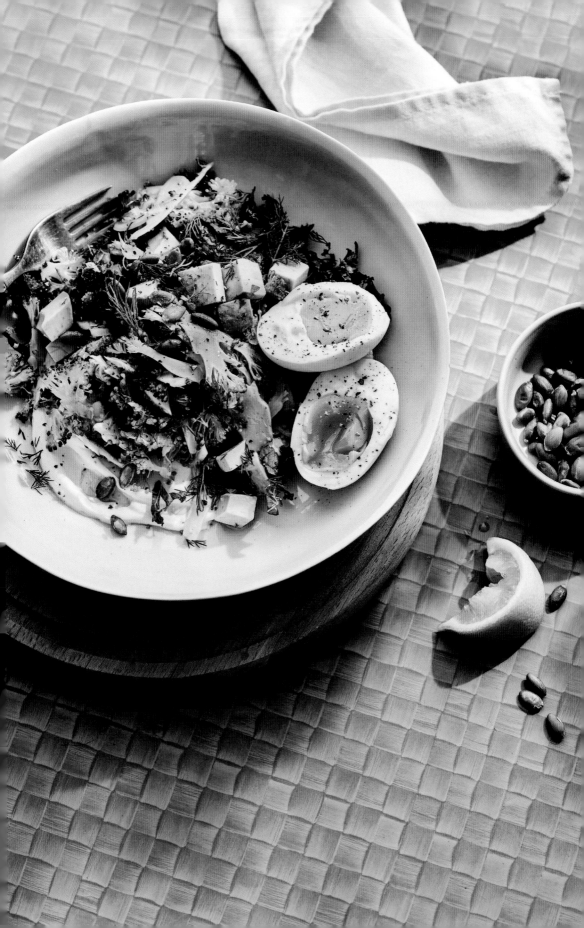

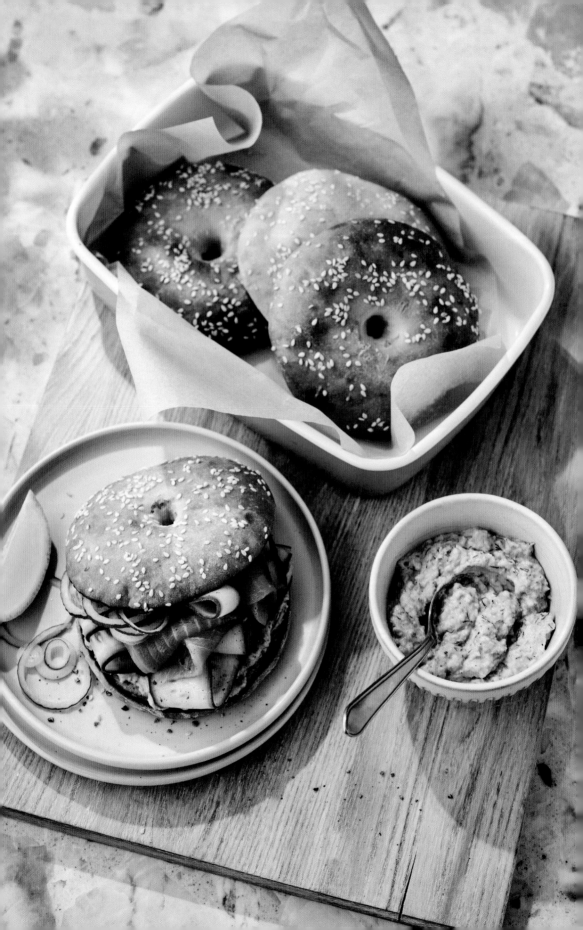

# Miracle Bagels

Yes, it's a SuperFastDiet phenomenon! Here is the miracle bagel, our just-as-delicious version of everyone's favourite brunch treat without the high-calorie tag. Make a double batch and keep them in the freezer for bagel indulgence whenever the brunch vibe hits you. Add some Everything Bagel Seasoning (see page 208) if you're wanting the whole American diner experience.

175 g (1¼ cups) self-raising flour, plus 1½ tablespoons for kneading
1 teaspoon sea salt flakes
310 g (1¼ cups) low-fat natural yoghurt

**TO SERVE**
1 avocado
60 g (¼ cup) low-fat natural yoghurt
1 tablespoon finely chopped dill
1 Lebanese cucumber, sliced into ribbons with a vegetable peeler
100 g smoked salmon slices
¼ small red onion, finely sliced

Preheat the oven to 180°C. Line a baking tray with baking paper.

Add the flour and salt to a bowl with 250 g (1 cup) of the yoghurt. Mix together with a wooden spoon or spatula until the mixture forms a shaggy dough. Continue to add the yoghurt as needed to just help bring the dough together. (It will depend on the moisture level of the yoghurt.) Sprinkle a little of the extra 1½ tablespoons of flour onto your work surface and knead the dough by hand for 5 minutes until soft and elastic. Sprinkle with the remaining flour as needed. Divide the dough into four and shape into balls. Use your finger to pierce a hole in the middle of each dough ball. Shape into a bagel shape, pulling and flattening as needed.

Place the dough on the prepared tray, then bake in the oven for 20 minutes until the bagels are golden on top. Carefully use tongs to flip the bagels over and continue baking for another 10 minutes until golden brown on the other side. Remove from the oven and allow to cool on a wire rack.

Mash the avocado and yoghurt together with a pinch each of salt and freshly ground black pepper, then stir in the dill.

Slice the bagels in half and toast them in the toaster, or in a frying pan over medium heat for a few minutes.

To assemble the bagels, on the bottom half, spread with the avocado mix, then top with the cucumber, the smoked salmon slices and the onion. Add the bagel top and serve.

---
### BOOST

⌃ Spray the bagels lightly with olive oil spray and sprinkle over 2 teaspoons of sesame seeds before baking. Extra 15 calories per serve.

---

**SERVES**
4

**PREP**
20 minutes

**COOK**
25 minutes

**CALS PER SERVE**
298

**ENTERTAINING**

# Herby Olive Frittata To Go

Start your day with an intense green hit. You can bake this frittata in advance and have brunch sorted for the whole week, mixing it up with salads and ham on the side for a super filling daily brunch, all good to go!

2 teaspoons extra-virgin olive oil

1 onion, finely diced

3 garlic cloves, finely sliced

6 free-range eggs

¾ cup firmly packed, finely chopped flat-leaf parsley

¾ cup firmly packed, finely chopped coriander

¼ cup firmly packed, finely chopped dill

1 cup firmly packed, finely shredded kale leaves

15 green olives, pitted and finely chopped

50 g (½ cup) finely shredded parmesan (a Microplane works well for this!)

**TO SERVE**

2 cups mixed lettuce leaves

125 g sliced ham (4 slices)

1 lemon, sliced into wedges

Preheat the oven to 180°C.

Place the olive oil in a large ovenproof frying pan (see note) over medium–high heat. Once hot, add the onion and garlic and cook for 5 minutes, stirring, until fragrant and golden. Turn off the heat and set aside.

Add the eggs, 1 teaspoon of salt and ¼ teaspoon of freshly ground black pepper to a mixing bowl and whisk well to combine. Add the parsley, coriander, dill, kale, olives, parmesan and the cooked onion and garlic and stir well to incorporate.

The frying pan should still be lightly greased from cooking the onion and garlic, so tip the frittata mixture into the pan and place over medium heat. Cook for 4 minutes, until the egg is set around the sides. Transfer to the oven and bake for 10 minutes until the frittata is browned around the edges and set in the middle.

Once cooked, remove from the oven and allow to cool completely before carefully removing from the pan and cutting into quarters.

Serve each slice with the lettuce, a slice of ham and a lemon wedge to squeeze over the lot.

## Notes

» If you don't own an ovenproof frying pan, transfer the frittata mixture into an oven-safe non-stick dish before baking.

» To freeze, divide the frittata into portions, then wrap first in baking paper, then plastic wrap. Freeze for up to 3 months. When ready to eat, thaw in the fridge overnight and warm up in the oven or microwave before serving.

| SERVES | PREP | COOK | CALS PER SERVE | GLUTEN FREE |
|---|---|---|---|---|
| 4 | 10 minutes | 20 minutes | 292 | |

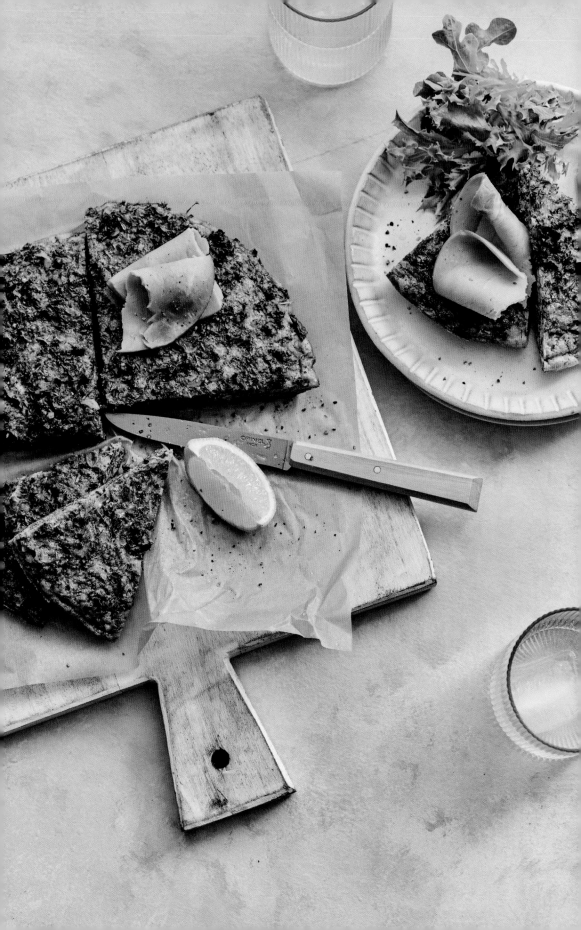

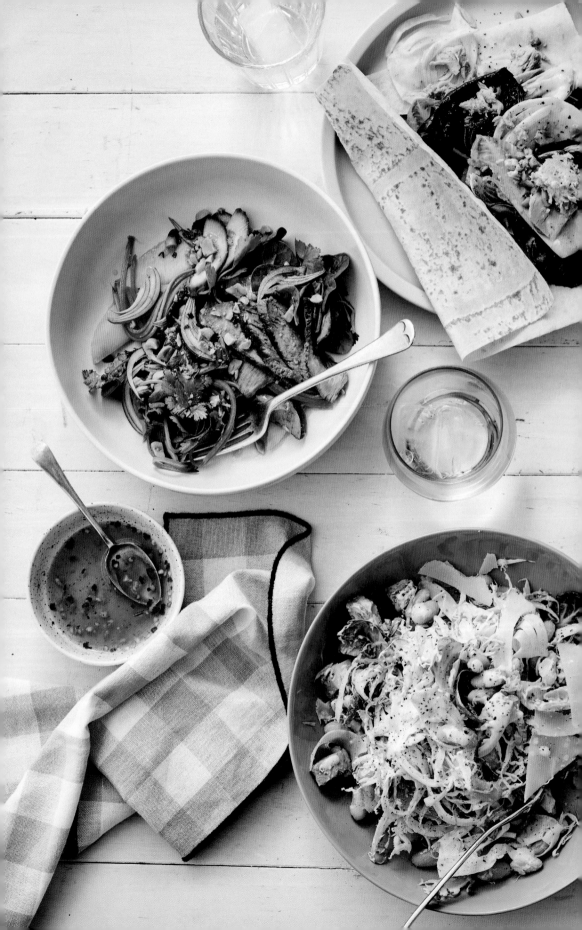

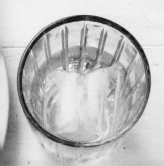

# Lunch

Lunch may well become your fave meal of the day as you savour every mouthful of these delicious recipes. You can have your meal at your usual lunchtime, or as dinner or even breakfast – in fact, whenever you want to fit it into your eating window and calorie allowance.

Finding nutritious and delicious lunch options can often be a challenge, especially if you're looking for low-calorie options that are easy to take to work. These mouthwatering lunch recipes are designed to fuel your body and keep you feeling satisfied throughout the day without compromising on taste.

Who knew low-cal eating could taste this good?

# 3-Minute Red Curry Noodles

Oh yes we did! While 3-minute noodles are notoriously heavy in saturated fats, we have the perfect, healthier solution that keeps all the flavour but drops the cals. Also, this dish is stacked with juicy prawns and fresh veg to make it extra filling. This recipe makes 4 x 500 ml jars. If you'd like to tote one to work, prepare a jar in the morning and when you're ready for lunch, simply add boiling water – 3 quick minutes later you'll be feasting!

150 g instant rice noodles (see note)

200 g small, shelled and deveined cooked prawns

1 head bok choy, roughly chopped

250 g shiitake mushrooms, finely sliced

1 carrot, shredded

4 spring onions, finely chopped

2 tablespoons red curry paste

1 teaspoon chicken stock powder

120 ml coconut milk

80 ml (⅓ cup) tamari or soy sauce

Divide all the ingredients between four 500 ml jars, airtight containers or serving bowls.

When ready to eat, just add 500 ml (2 cups) of boiling water. Cover for 3–4 minutes for the noodles to soften, then eat!

Premade jars will last in the fridge for up to 5 days.

**Note** You can find instant rice noodles in the health food section of your supermarket or grocer. It may be easier to purchase instant noodles and discard the flavourings sachet.

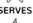

| SERVES | PREP | COOK | CALS PER SERVE | DAIRY FREE | 15 MINUTES OR LESS |
|---|---|---|---|---|---|
| 4 | 10 minutes | 3 minutes | 290 | | |

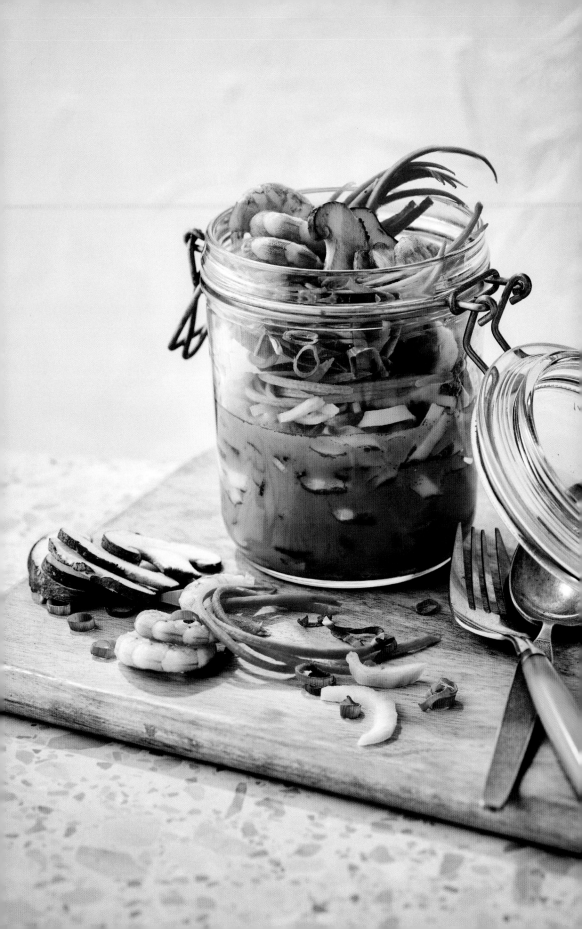

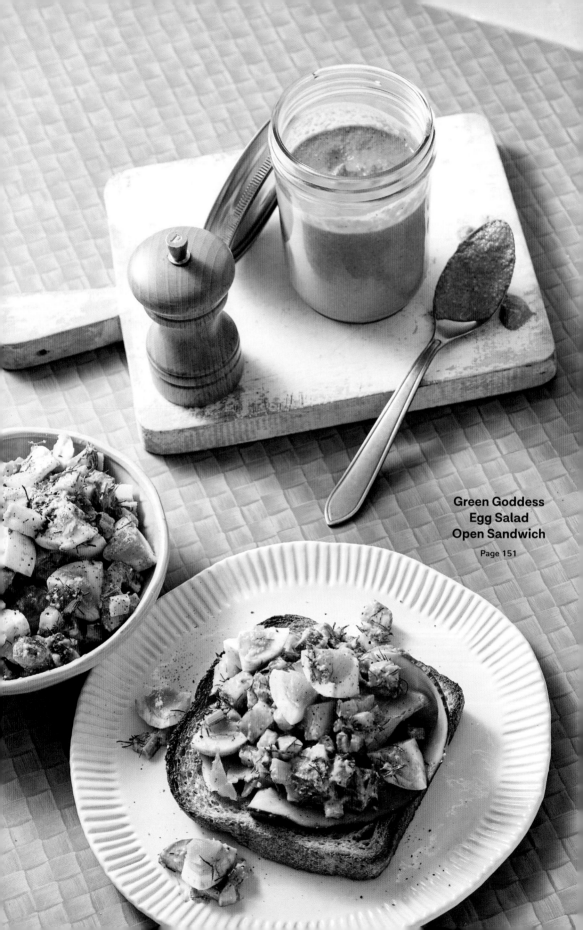

**Green Goddess
Egg Salad
Open Sandwich**

Page 151

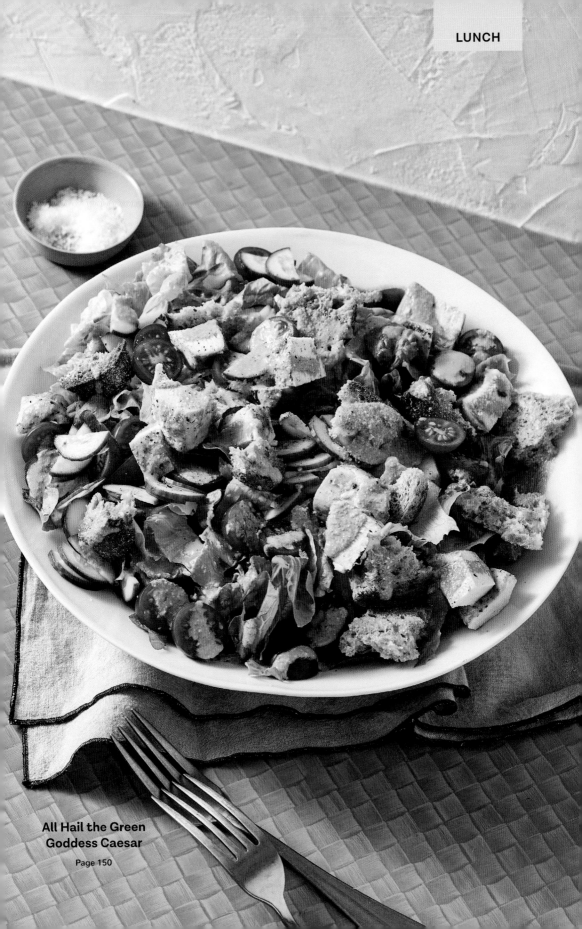

**All Hail the Green
Goddess Caesar**

Page 150

# All Hail the Green Goddess Caesar

Our green goddess dressing is truly divine, and it's high in veg and low in calories. You can use it in all your salads, although this caesar recipe rules. You can even spoon the dressing over roast veg or grilled protein too. There's nothing she can't magically transform. The amount of dressing you'll make here is 1½ cups, which is enough for this caesar salad plus the Green Goddess Egg Salad Open Sandwich opposite.

2 heads cos lettuce,
    roughly chopped
1 Lebanese cucumber, cut into
    5 mm half moons
200 g cherry tomatoes, halved
250 g store-bought cooked
    chicken breast, roughly
    chopped (see note)
4 slices wholemeal bread,
    toasted and chopped or
    torn into small pieces

**SUPERFAST GREEN
GODDESS DRESSING**

1 small golden shallot
40 g (¼ cup) raw cashews
20 g (1 cup) baby spinach leaves
1 bunch of basil, leaves picked
1 garlic clove, minced
Juice of 2 lemons
1 tablespoon extra-virgin
    olive oil
30 g (⅓ cup) grated parmesan
1 teaspoon sea salt flakes
¼ teaspoon freshly ground
    black pepper
1–4 tablespoons water

To make the dressing, add all the ingredients, except the water, to a blender and blitz on high until smooth and creamy, adding 1 tablespoon of the water at a time, as needed, to allow the sauce to blend.

Put the lettuce, cucumber, cherry tomatoes and chicken in a large bowl, then pour half the dressing (reserving the remaining for another time) over the top and toss to coat the salad.

Divide the salad between four bowls and top with the toasted 'croutons' to serve.

**Note** You can purchase pre-cooked roasted chicken breast in the deli section of the supermarket.

---

**BOOST**

⌃ Serve with 1 medium
    boiled egg. Extra 65
    calories per serve.

---

**SERVES**
4

**PREP**
20 minutes

**CALS PER
SERVE**
287

**20
MINUTES
OR LESS**

# Green Goddess Egg Salad Open Sandwich

Creamy egg salad sandwiches are delicious, but swapping out the mayo for the far lower-calorie SuperFast Green Goddess Dressing just makes sense, right? ... delicious, goddessy sense.

6 free-range eggs

2 Lebanese cucumbers, finely diced

3 celery stalks, finely diced

2 teaspoons dijon mustard

2 tablespoons finely chopped dill

½ quantity (¾ cup) SuperFast Green Goddess Dressing (opposite)

4 slices wholemeal bread, toasted

130 g finely sliced sliced ham (four slices)

Fill a medium saucepan with water and place over high heat. Once boiling, add the eggs and cook, undisturbed, for 8 minutes. Remove the eggs with a slotted spoon and run them under cool water until cool to the touch. Peel and finely chop.

Add the egg, cucumber, celery, mustard, dill and the dressing to a large bowl and toss to combine.

Divide the toast among four serving plates, top with the egg salad and a slice of ham and serve.

---

**BOOST**

» Serve as a closed sandwich with another slice of wholemeal bread on top. Extra 67 calories per serve.

---

**SERVES**
4

**PREP**
20 minutes

**COOK**
10 minutes

**CALS PER SERVE**
300

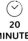
**20 MINUTES OR LESS**

# Peanut Tuna Wrap with Torn Leaves & Fennel

Perfect on a busy day, this tasty wrap can be whipped up in 10 minutes flat for a nutritious and delicious lunch. The vinaigrette can be used on any salad, so we recommend you make extra and keep it to elevate your next lunch – better put your name on it if that's in the work fridge. #toodelishtoresist

3 cups roughly torn radicchio leaves

2 heads witlof, leaves picked

1 small fennel bulb, finely sliced

30 g dry-roasted, unsalted peanuts, finely chopped

8 x 25 g store-bought mountain bread wraps (see notes)

360 g tuna chunks in spring water, drained

### VINAIGRETTE

2 teaspoons dijon mustard

1 teaspoon extra-virgin olive oil

2 teaspoons honey

Juice of 1 lemon

½ teaspoon sea salt flakes

¼ teaspoon freshly ground black pepper

To make the vinaigrette, put all the ingredients in a large bowl and mix to combine.

Add the radicchio, witlof, fennel and peanuts to the bowl and toss gently to coat in the dressing.

Divide the wraps between four serving plates, then fill with the dressed leaves and tuna. Wrap up and eat immediately.

## Notes

» Mountain bread wraps are commonly found in all major supermarkets in Australia. All variations are roughly 72 calories per wrap. If you cannot find these wraps in your supermarket, use any wrap or carbohydrate that adds up to 145 calories per serve.

» If you're preparing this meal in advance for lunches, keep the salad and tuna separate from the wrap until ready to eat.

## BOOST

⌃ Add a quarter of a medium avocado. Extra 65 calories per serve.

**SERVES**
4

**PREP**
10 minutes

**CALS PER SERVE**
303

**DAIRY FREE**

**15 MINUTES OR LESS**

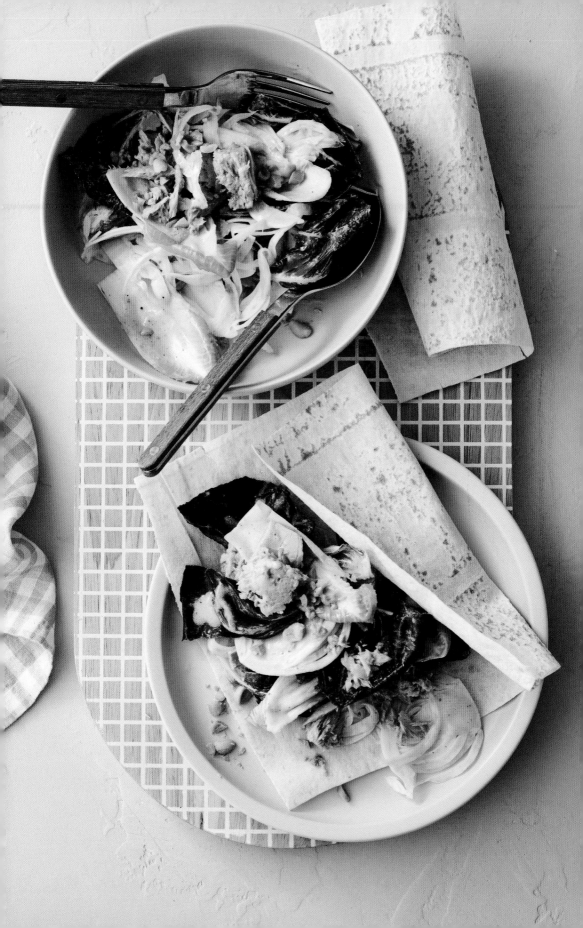

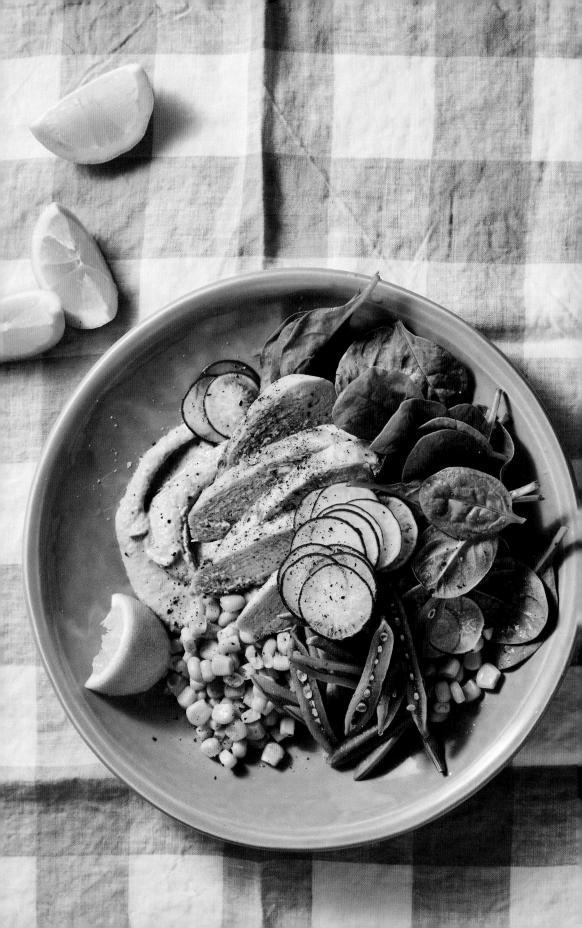

# Ultimate Chicken Power Bowls

This power bowl is the ultimate 10-minute lunch. It's an easy salad of chicken, raw veggies and store-bought staples, coated in creamy hummus – get ready to power through the afternoon!

500 g store-bought cooked chicken breast (see note)

6 radishes, finely sliced

100 g sugar snap peas, trimmed and halved

150 g (¾ cup) canned corn kernels, drained and rinsed

80 g (4 cups) baby spinach leaves

110 g (½ cup) hummus

½ teaspoon sea salt flakes

1 lemon, sliced into wedges

Divide the chicken, vegetables and hummus between four bowls. Season with the salt and some freshly ground black pepper, then squeeze the lemon wedges over the lot. Toss everything together to coat in the lemon juice and hummus, forming a creamy, zingy dressing.

**Note** You can purchase pre-cooked roasted chicken breast in the deli section of the supermarket.

## BOOST

≫ Serve with ¼ cup cooked quinoa (extra 57 calories per serve) and/or 1 tablespoon dry-roasted pumpkin seeds (extra 63 calories per serve).

**SERVES**
4

**PREP**
10 minutes

**CALS PER SERVE**
300

**GLUTEN FREE**

**DAIRY FREE**

**15 MINUTES OR LESS**

# Winter Slaw with Sesame Dressing

Seasonal produce becomes a winter slaw delight when coated in nutty sesame dressing. Add some cannellini beans and creamy avocado and you've got yourself a hearty and super nutritious lunchtime treat.

## WINTER SLAW

300 g brussels sprouts,
    shredded (see notes)
¼ green cabbage, finely
    shredded
1 small fennel bulb, finely sliced
2 x 400 g cans cannellini beans,
    drained and rinsed
    (yields 3 cups of beans)
1 small avocado, diced

## SESAME DRESSING

2 tablespoons sesame seeds
    (see notes)
1 tablespoon extra-virgin
    olive oil
1 teaspoon dijon mustard
20 g parmesan, finely shaved
Juice of 1 lemon
1 teaspoon sea salt flakes
Pinch of freshly ground
    black pepper

To make the sesame dressing, place a large non-stick frying pan over medium heat. Add the sesame seeds and cook, tossing, for 5 minutes, until lightly golden. Tip into a mortar and pestle and grind until fine.

Put the ground sesame seeds in a jar or bowl with the remaining dressing ingredients and shake or stir to combine. Add 1–3 teaspoons of water if needed, to make the dressing runny enough to pour. Set aside.

Add all the ingredients for the winter slaw to a large bowl and toss to combine. Pour the dressing over the top and toss gently to coat the salad. Divide between four bowls to serve.

## Notes

» The brussels sprouts, cabbage and fennel are easily sliced using a mandoline.
» To prepare this for lunches to take to school or work, put the dressing in the bottom of containers or large jars. Add the beans so they sit in the dressing, then pile the slaw on top, followed lastly by the avocado. Squeeze some lemon juice over the avocado to stop it from going brown, then place on the lid. When ready to eat, dump the salad into a bowl and toss everything together to coat in the dressing.
» You can replace the sesame seeds with 1 tablespoon of tahini and just mix with the lemon juice and some warm water until you form a runny dressing.

**SERVES**
4

**PREP**
15 minutes

**COOK**
5 minutes

**CALS PER SERVE**
306

**GLUTEN FREE**

**VEGETARIAN**

**20 MINUTES OR LESS**

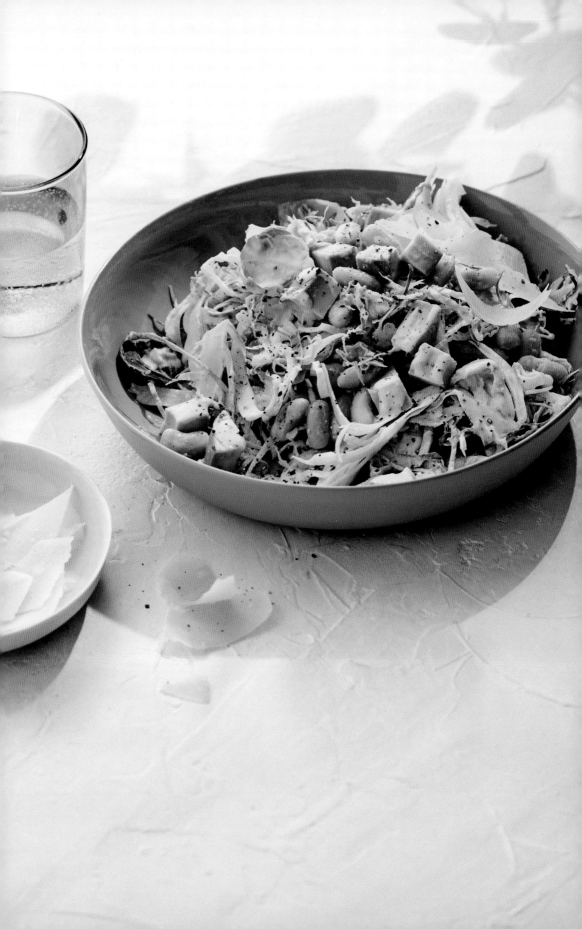

# Reuben Club Sandwich

There's proof right here that you don't have to give up the gourmet good stuff with SuperFastDiet. We've managed to pack in all the saucy, decadent fun you'd expect from a classic reuben at only 310 calories a serve. We know. Too good.

8 slices rye bread, toasted

145 g (1 cup) store-bought sauerkraut

200 g sliced beef pastrami

3 cups shredded iceberg lettuce

2 tomatoes, sliced

1 small red onion, finely sliced

**RUSSIAN DRESSING**

95 g (⅓ cup) low-fat natural yoghurt

2 teaspoons tomato sauce

2 teaspoons horseradish cream

1 teaspoon worcestershire sauce

1 small garlic clove, minced

Pinch of smoked paprika

Add all the dressing ingredients to a bowl and mix well to combine.

Spread each piece of toast with Russian dressing. Top four of the slices with the sauerkraut, pastrami, lettuce, tomato and red onion. Place the other piece of toast on top to make four sandwiches, then serve.

**SERVES**
4

**PREP**
10 minutes

**CALS PER SERVE**
310

**15 MINUTES OR LESS**

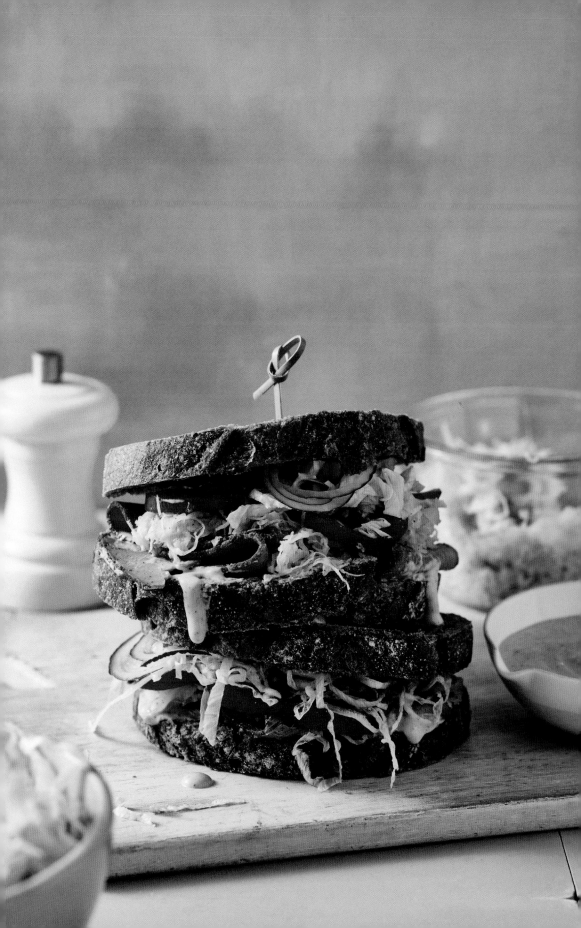

# Chickpea Nori Hand Salad

Nom nom, nori. And so handy to have ... er, on hand for busy days.
(You've got to hand it to us – three 'hand' references in a row there!)
Nori is actually a brilliant alternative to higher-calorie breads and rolls
and it's a great vehicle to fill up with all the good stuff. Let's give good
old nori a hand. (Okay, we'll stop now.)

8 sheets nori, cut into quarters

3 cups shredded iceberg lettuce

1 carrot, shredded

½ avocado, sliced or diced

1 tablespoon sriracha, to serve

**CRUSHED CHICKPEAS**

400 g (2 cups) canned
   chickpeas, drained and rinsed

1 tablespoon sriracha

1 tablespoon mayonnaise

1 tablespoon tamari
   or soy sauce

½ teaspoon sea salt flakes

Pinch of ground turmeric

For the crushed chickpeas, place the chickpeas in a large
bowl and mash with a potato masher or fork until mostly
crushed. Add the remaining crushed chickpea ingredients
and mix until combined.

Divide the nori, lettuce, carrot, avocado and the crushed
chickpeas between four plates to serve and top with some
sriracha to finish. Diners can fill their sheets of nori just
before eating, so they don't become soggy.

---

## BOOST

» Add 95 g (½ cup) cooked
  jasmine rice. Extra 119
  calories per serve.

---

**SERVES**
4

**PREP**
15 minutes

**CALS PER
SERVE**
222

**VEGETARIAN**

**15
MINUTES
OR LESS**

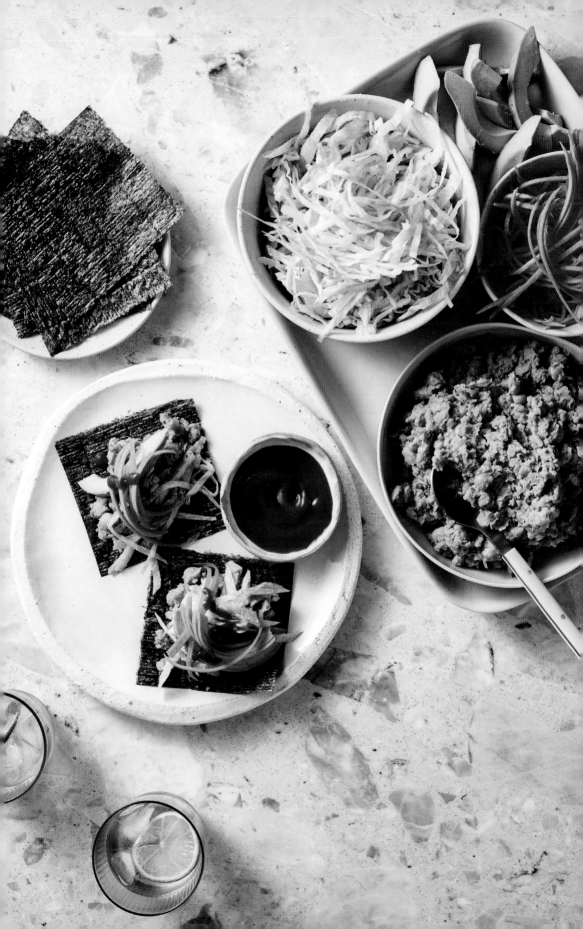

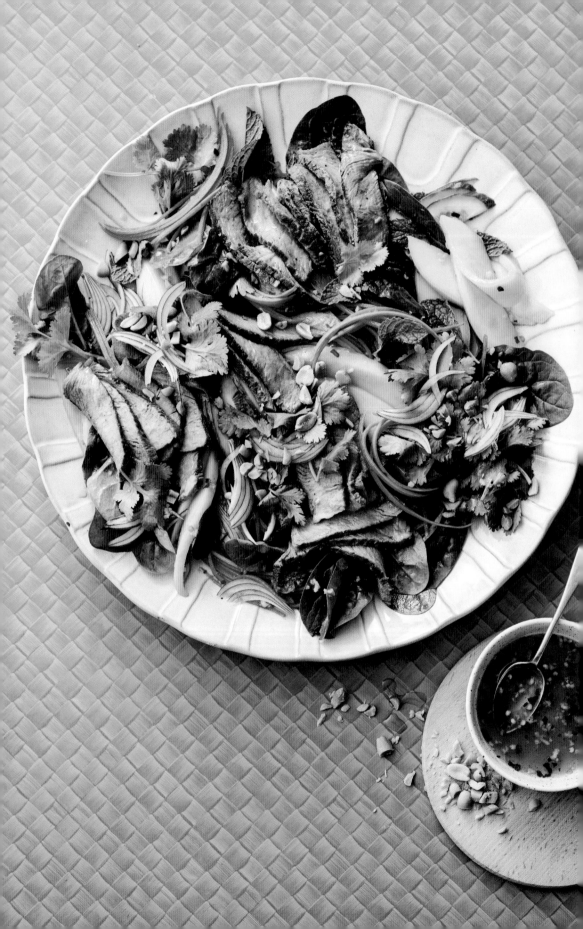

# Thai Beef, Mango & Peanut Salad

Tropical delights at lunchtime anyone? This classic Thai beef salad
absolutely zings with the addition of juicy fresh mango. Throw in some
crushed peanuts and enjoy a little mind holiday on us.

500 g lean beef steak
½ teaspoon sea salt flakes
½ teaspoon extra-virgin olive oil

**DRESSING**
2 tablespoons fish sauce
1½ tablespoons rice wine
  vinegar
Juice of 1 lime
1 tablespoon honey
1 small garlic clove,
  finely minced
Pinch of dried chilli flakes

**MANGO & PEANUT SALAD**
1 carrot, shredded
1 Lebanese cucumber, finely
  sliced into half moons
¼ red onion, finely sliced
60 g (3 cups) baby spinach
  leaves
1 cup coriander leaves,
  roughly chopped
1 cup mint leaves,
  roughly chopped
30 g (¼ cup) roasted, unsalted
  peanuts, chopped
1 ripe mango, sliced

Season the beef on both sides with the sea salt flakes.

Heat the olive oil in a large non-stick frying pan over high
heat. Once hot, add the steak and cook for 3–4 minutes
on each side. Remove from the heat and transfer to a plate
to rest for 5 minutes, then slice finely.

Add all the dressing ingredients to a jar and shake
to combine.

For the mango and peanut salad, add all the ingredients to
a large bowl and toss to combine. Drizzle with the dressing
and toss to coat.

Divide the salad between four plates and serve with the
sliced steak.

**Notes** To keep this salad for leftovers, keep the dressing
in the jar and only pour it over the salad right before you eat.

|  |  |  |  |  |  |  |
|---|---|---|---|---|---|---|
| **SERVES** 4 | **PREP** 10 minutes | **COOK** 10 minutes | **CALS PER SERVE** 312 | **GLUTEN FREE** | **DAIRY FREE** | **20 MINUTES OR LESS** |

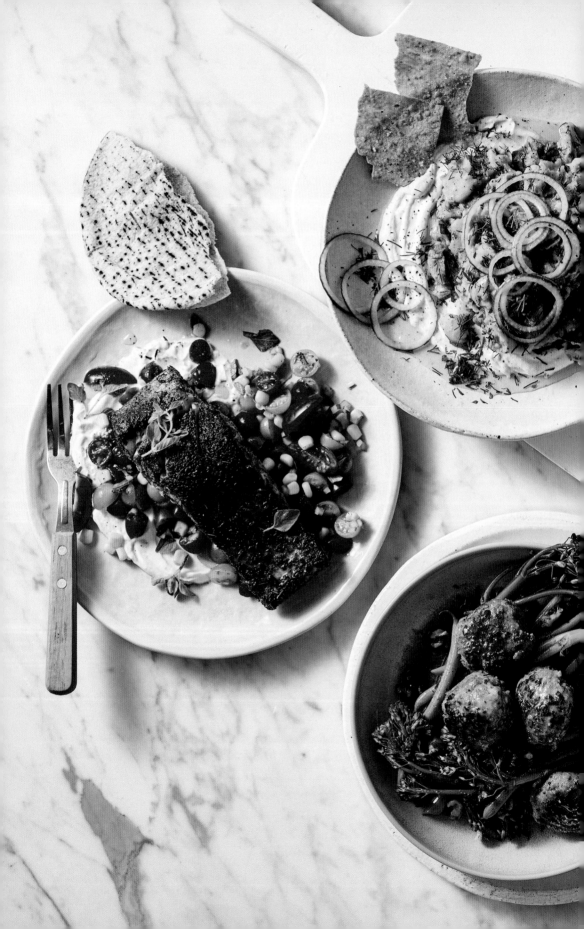

# Mains

These aren't just main meals, they're party-level hearty. You'll be amazed how full and satisfied you'll feel after eating them – and how decadent they taste for such low calories.

Whether you're looking for a quick and easy (but super yum) weeknight dinner, or a special-occasion meal, these recipes are sensational!

With so much colourful variety to choose from you'll never be left wondering what to eat – only how to hide the leftovers in the fridge from the fam so you can have more tomorrow.

# BBQ Chicken Steaks with Chargrilled Vegetables

These juicy and super tasty barbecued chicken steaks are perfection served with the smoky chargrilled vegetables. Add some Roasted Garlic Cream (page 220) and you've got the perfect solution for weeknight dinners or entertaining friends.

2 red capsicums, deseeded
    and sliced into 5 cm pieces
2 corn cobs, husk removed
2 zucchini, sliced into ribbons
1 red onion, sliced into
    1 cm rings
1 bunch of asparagus, woody
    ends trimmed
1½ tablespoons extra-virgin
    olive oil
Sea salt flakes
2 tablespoons oregano leaves
125 g (½ cup) Roasted Garlic
    Cream (page 220) or low-fat
    natural yoghurt, to serve

**BBQ CHICKEN**
600 g chicken breast fillets –
    2 x 300 g breasts sliced in
    half horizontally to make
    4 thin steaks
2 teaspoons extra-virgin olive oil
2 teaspoons smoked paprika
2 teaspoons ground cumin
½ teaspoon sea salt flakes
300 g (1 cup) Smoky BBQ Sauce
    (page 224)

For the BBQ chicken, place the chicken breast fillets in a large bowl. Drizzle with the olive oil and season with the paprika, cumin, salt and some freshly ground black pepper. Toss to coat well.

Preheat a barbecue grill plate to high, or heat a cast-iron chargrill pan over high heat on the stovetop.

Place the chicken on the barbecue or in the chargrill pan and cook for 2 minutes on each side. Baste the chicken with the barbecue sauce, flip and cook for 1 minute. Baste the other side and flip again, cooking for another 1 minute. Transfer to a plate for resting.

While the chicken is resting, place the veggies in a large bowl and drizzle with the olive oil and season with a pinch of sea salt flakes, ¼ teaspoon freshly ground black pepper and the oregano. Place on the barbecue or in the chargrill pan and cook for 10 minutes, tossing each vegetable until lightly charred all over and tender.

Slice the corn thickly, then divide the vegetables and BBQ chicken between four plates. Serve with a dollop of roasted garlic cream.

| SERVES | PREP | COOK | CALS PER SERVE | GLUTEN FREE | ENTERTAINING |
|---|---|---|---|---|---|
| 4 | 10 minutes | 30 minutes | 391 | | |

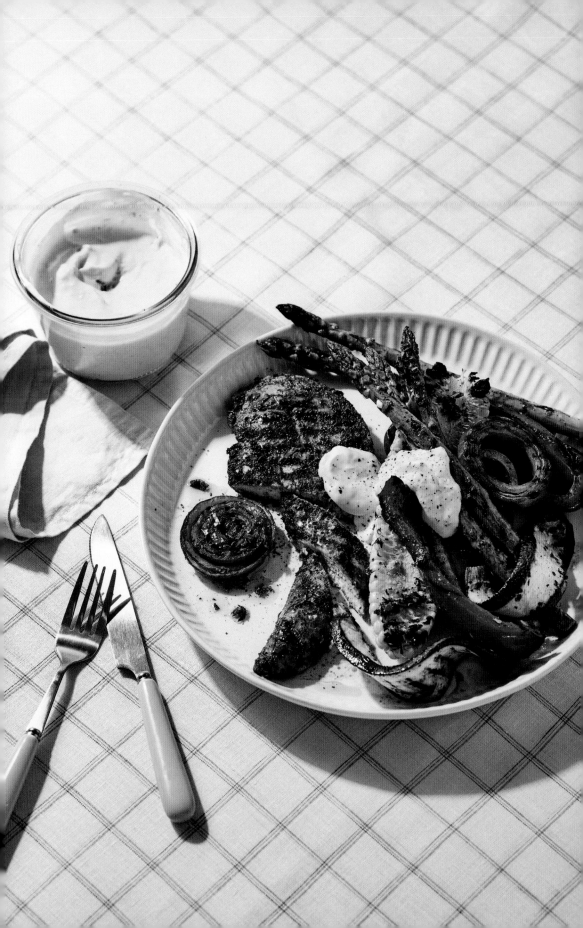

# Resting Roast Chicken on Ratatouille Bed

A one-pot resting stop to sit and savour all the rich and filling flavours of French cuisine. This dish is so wholesome and satisfying you'll find it hard to believe it's only 400 calories a serve ... and you may just need une sieste yourself after this hearty meal. Zzzz.

600 g chicken thigh fillets, trimmed of excess fat
Sea salt flakes
1 teaspoon extra-virgin olive oil
1 tablespoon apple cider vinegar
8 garlic cloves, finely sliced
10 green olives, pitted and roughly chopped
1 bunch of oregano, leaves picked
2 zucchini, cut into 2 cm slices
3 roma tomatoes, quartered
1 red onion, roughly chopped
2 red capsicums, deseeded and chopped into 2 cm chunks
250 ml (1 cup) chicken stock

Preheat the oven to 180°C.

Season the chicken thighs on both sides with sea salt flakes and some freshly ground black pepper. Heat the olive oil in a large cast-iron ovenproof pot over medium–high heat. Once the oil is hot, add the chicken to the pot and cook for 4 minutes on each side until golden brown and cooked through. Remove the chicken from the pot and set aside.

Add the vinegar, garlic, olives and oregano to the pot and cook for 1 minute, scraping off any chicken bits from the bottom of the pot. Add the zucchini, tomatoes, onion, capsicum, stock and a pinch each of salt and freshly ground black pepper. Bring to a simmer, then remove from the heat. Place a lid on the pot, then transfer to the oven and bake for 20 minutes.

In the last 5 minutes of cooking time, nestle the chicken thighs (and any juice) into the pot. Return to the oven and bake for another 5 minutes, until the chicken has warmed through.

Divide the chicken and vegetables between four plates and serve.

---

## BOOST

⌃ Serve with 1 slice (50 g) of toasted, crusty sourdough bread to mop up all the juices. Extra 180 calories per serve.

---

 **SERVES**
4

 **PREP**
10 minutes

 **COOK**
35 minutes

 **CALS PER SERVE**
401

**GLUTEN FREE**

 **DAIRY FREE**

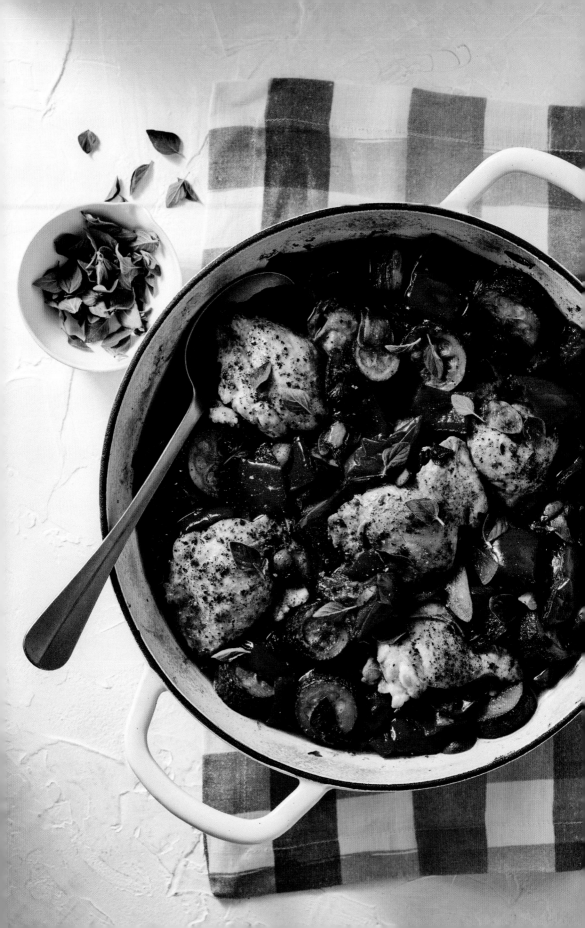

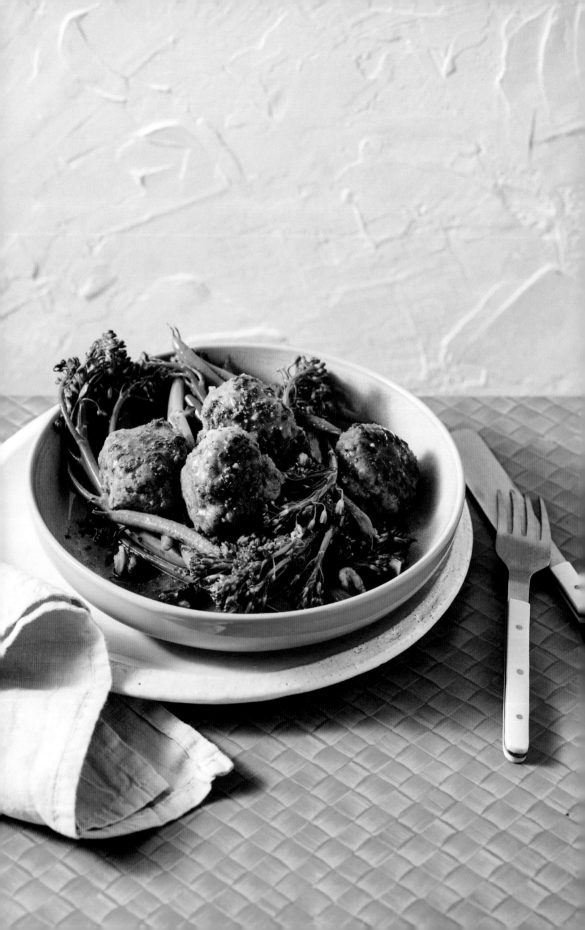

# Lemon Caper Chicken Meatballs with Walnut Greens

Woohoo! What a delicious caper these meatballs are – and decadent too!
This dish has all the trimmings: cheese, butter, olive oil, nuts ... and yet it
still comes in at only 402 calories per serve. We know, right?

500 g lean chicken mince

1 free-range egg

30 g (½ cup) panko breadcrumbs

¼ cup oregano leaves,
    finely chopped, plus extra
    to garnish

2 tablespoons capers in vinegar,
    drained

3 garlic cloves, minced

30 g parmesan, finely grated

Zest and juice of 1 lemon

2 teaspoons extra-virgin olive oil

2 teaspoons apple cider vinegar

250 ml (1 cup) chicken stock

20 g salted butter

**WALNUT GREENS**

2 teaspoons extra-virgin olive oil

200 g green beans, trimmed

1 bunch of broccolini, thick
    stalks sliced in half
    lengthways

2 tablespoons roughly chopped
    walnuts

### BOOST

⚠ Roast 600 g potatoes in
the oven with 1 teaspoon
of olive oil. Extra 88
calories per serve.

To make the meatballs, put the mince, egg, breadcrumbs,
oregano, capers, garlic, parmesan and lemon zest in a bowl.
Use your hands to combine the mixture really well. Scoop
up 1 tablespoon amounts, roughly shape into meatballs and
place on a plate. (Note: these are sticky and that's okay!
Don't add flour as it will dry them out.)

Heat the olive oil in a frying pan over medium–high heat.
Once hot, add the meatballs and cook for 1–2 minutes,
tossing, to brown the outside. Reduce the heat to medium
and continue cooking and tossing regularly for 4 minutes,
until mostly cooked. Remove from the pan and set aside.

For the walnut greens, add the olive oil to the same pan
still over medium–high. Once hot, add the green beans and
broccolini. Cook, tossing for 3 minutes, until bright green.
Add the walnuts and continue tossing for 3 minutes, until
the walnuts are golden and the greens are tender. Tip into
a bowl and cover with foil to keep warm.

Add the vinegar to the pan and cook for 1 minute, using
a wooden spoon or spatula to scrape off any bits from
the bottom. Add the the stock, butter, lemon juice and
extra oregano and cook, stirring, for 2 minutes until well
combined. Return the meatballs to the pan and continue
to simmer for 2–3 minutes, until cooked through.

Divide the meatballs and walnut greens between four
plates, spoon the butter sauce from the pan over the top
and serve.

**SERVES**
4

**PREP**
10 minutes

**COOK**
20 minutes

**CALS PER SERVE**
402

**30 MINUTES OR LESS**

# Chipotle Chicken Tacos with Green Tomato Salsa

On a fasting day, but you've invited friends around for dinner? We've got you! This is THE ultimate low-calorie entertaining meal. At only 410 calories per serve, you'll be feasting without breaking the calorie bank! Fantástico!

2 teaspoons extra-virgin olive oil
500 g chicken thigh fillets
¼ teaspoon sea salt flakes
½ white onion, finely diced
4 garlic cloves, minced
2 teaspoons ground cumin
2 teaspoons apple cider vinegar
2 tablespoons chipotle chillies
 in adobo sauce
250 ml (1 cup) chicken stock
8 x 25 g mini flour or gluten-free
 tortillas, warmed
125 g (½ cup) Roasted Garlic
 Cream (page 220) or low-fat
 natural yoghurt
4 leaves baby cos
½ cup cherry tomatoes, halved

**GREEN TOMATO SALSA**
450 g green tomatoes,
 quartered
4 garlic cloves, unpeeled
½ white onion, finely diced
2 cups coriander leaves,
 plus extra to serve
Juice of 1 lime
½ teaspoon sea salt flakes

Preheat the oven grill to 200°C.

Place 1 teaspoon of the olive oil in a deep, heavy-based saucepan over medium–high heat. Season the chicken thighs on both sides with the salt and ¼ teaspoon freshly ground black pepper, then place in the pan. Cook for 4 minutes on each side until cooked through. Set aside on a plate to rest for 5 minutes, then shred the meat using two forks.

Reduce the heat to medium and add the onion and the remaining oil to the pan. Cook, stirring, for 3 minutes until golden, adding a dash of water if needed. Add the garlic and cumin and cook for 1 minute until fragrant. Add the vinegar and stir it through for 30 seconds, scraping any chicken bits from the bottom of the pot. Add the chipotle chillies and stock and stir to combine. Add the shredded chicken and any resting juices. Bring to a simmer and cook for 20 minutes, reducing the liquid by half, while you prepare the salsa.

For the green tomato salsa, place the tomatoes on a large baking tray with the garlic. Place under the oven grill and cook for 20 minutes, until the tomatoes are blackened slightly and the garlic is tender. Transfer the tomatoes to a food processor. Squeeze the garlic flesh out of the skins and add to the food processor, with the onion, coriander, lime juice, salt and ¼ teaspoon freshly ground black pepper. Blitz to a chunky paste. Alternatively, finely chop all the ingredients and mix to combine.

Serve the shredded chipotle chicken on a platter in the middle of the table with the green tomato salsa, warmed tortillas, garlic cream, cos leaves and baby tomatoes.

 **SERVES** 4
 **PREP** 10 minutes
 **COOK** 35 minutes
 **CALS PER SERVE** 415
 **GLUTEN FREE**
 **ENTERTAINING**

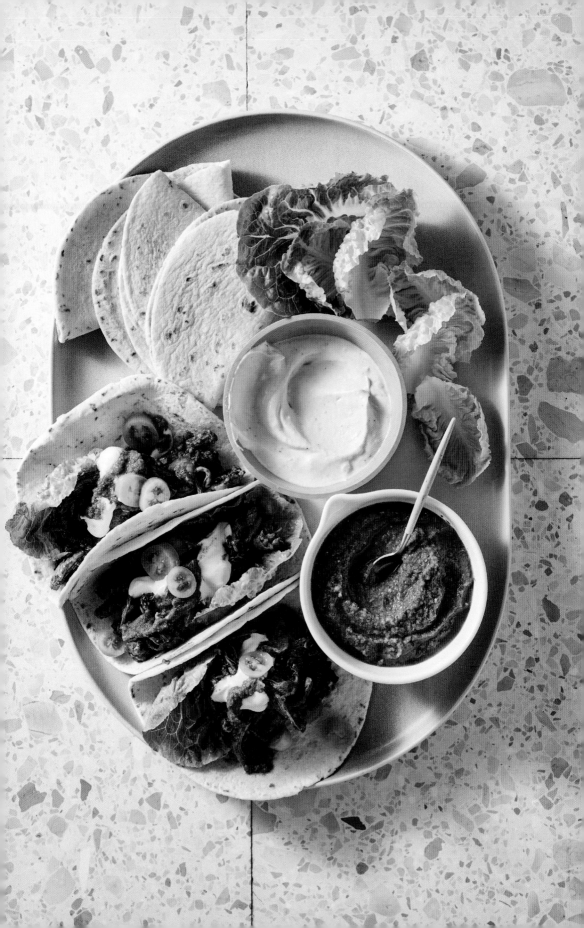

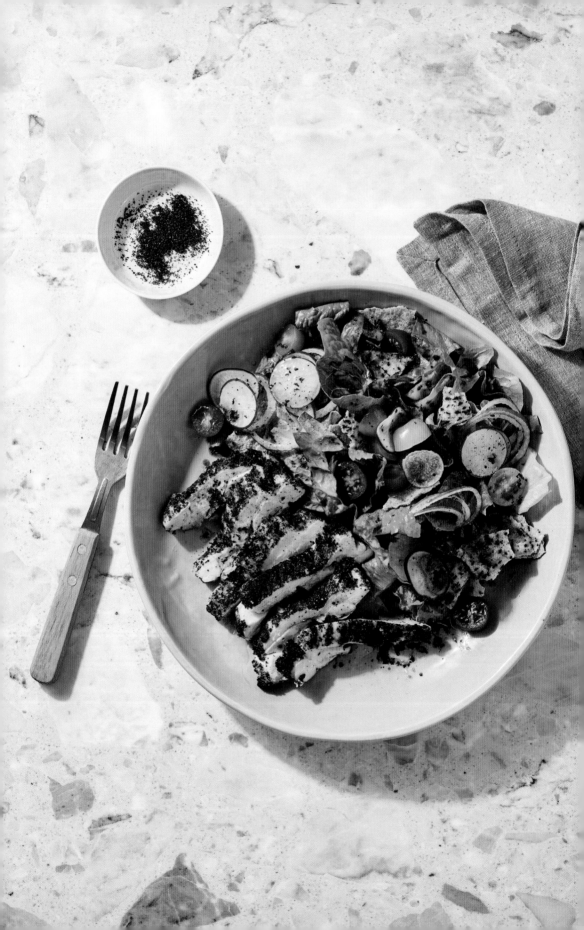

# Chargrilled Sumac Chicken with Not-So-Fattoush Salad

Okay, SFD super secret alert: using the barbecue to grill protein is one of our best hacks to keep calories low. You don't need oil, the meat stays tender and you get all that sensationally smoky chargrilled flavour. Plus you get to cook outside in glorious nature and have a little me time. #justchilling

2 large pita breads
600 g chicken thigh fillets
1 tablespoon sumac
1 teaspoon sea salt flakes
4 cups roughly chopped
    cos lettuce
250 g cherry tomatoes, halved
½ red onion, finely sliced
6 radishes, finely sliced

**LEMON, POMEGRANATE & MINT DRESSING**

Juice of 1 lemon
1 teaspoon pomegranate
    molasses
1 teaspoon dried mint
1 tablespoon extra-virgin
    olive oil

Preheat the oven to 180°C and a barbecue grill plate to high (see note).

Place the pita bread pieces across two large baking trays and bake in the oven for 15 minutes, until golden brown, then tear into pieces.

Add the chicken to a large bowl and sprinkle with the sumac, sea salt flakes and ¼ teaspoon freshly ground black pepper. Toss to coat well.

Once the barbecue is hot, place the chicken on the grill and cook for 6 minutes each side, or until cooked through. Slice.

Add all the ingredients for the dressing to a large bowl and mix to combine. Add the lettuce, cherry tomatoes, onion and radish to the bowl, then toss gently to coat everything in the dressing. Add the toasted pita and toss again to combine.

Divide the not-so-fattoush salad and barbecued chicken between four plates and serve.

**Note** You could also cook the chicken in a chargrill pan on the stovetop over high heat.

--- BOOST ---

⌃ Add 1 tablespoon (15 g) of roughly chopped, roasted almonds. Extra 90 calories per serve.

| SERVES | PREP | COOK | CALS PER SERVE | DAIRY FREE | 30 MINUTES OR LESS | ENTERTAINING |
|---|---|---|---|---|---|---|
| 4 | 10 minutes | 15 minutes | 389 | | | |

# Lemony Spring Chicken Soup

You'll feel like a spring chicken when you devour this soup for the soul. Packed with a bounty of fresh veg, garlic, lemon and some pasta and cheese for good measure, you'll have a spring in your step for the rest of the day!

1 tablespoon extra-virgin olive oil

400 g chicken breast fillets

½ teaspoon sea salt flakes

1 leek, finely sliced

3 celery stalks, diced

4 garlic cloves, finely sliced

2 litres chicken stock (or 2 litres of water with 2 teaspoons of chicken stock paste)

80 g short pasta, such as penne or spirals

2 cups shredded silverbeet or kale

110 g (¾ cup) frozen peas

Juice of 1 lemon

40 g parmesan, shaved

Heat 2 teaspoons of the olive oil in a large, heavy-based saucepan over medium heat. Season the chicken breast with a pinch of salt and ¼ teaspoon freshly ground black pepper and place in the pan. Cook for 5 minutes, then flip and add 125 ml (½ cup) water to the pot, then cover with a lid. Cook for 7–10 minutes, until the chicken breast is cooked through. Remove the chicken from the pan and slice finely.

Place the pan back over medium heat – there shouldn't be any water left, if there is, discard it. Add the remaining 2 teaspoons of olive oil, leek, celery and garlic and cook for 3 minutes until softened and fragrant. Add the chicken stock and sea salt, bring to the boil, then add the pasta. Cook the pasta for 2 minutes less than the packet instructions say, then add the shredded chicken, silverbeet and frozen peas to the pot. Continue cooking for a further 2 minutes.

Remove the pan from the heat and squeeze the lemon juice in, then add most of the parmesan and stir it through.

Divide the soup between four bowls and garnish with any remaining parmesan and some freshly ground black pepper.

**Note** To freeze, divide the soup into portions and place in airtight containers or jars. Freeze for up to 3 months.

## BOOST

» Fry 80 g of diced bacon before the vegetables to add a great smoky flavour to your soup. Extra 107 calories per serve.

 **SERVES** 4

 **PREP** 10 minutes

 **COOK** 30 minutes

 **CALS PER SERVE** 403

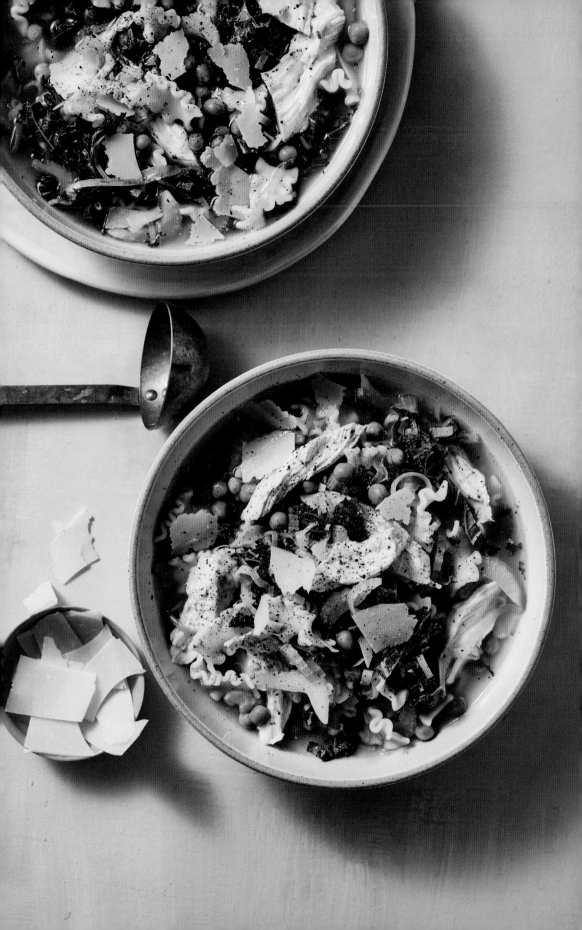

# Creamy Herby Steak Skewers with Grilled Broccoli

The humble combo of steak and broccoli just got a makeover – and you're about to fall in love! We've gone heavy on the condiments using creamy Homemade Labne (page 222) and herby Salsa Verde (page 227). Easy to make, impossible not to swoon.

650 g beef steak, such as scotch fillet, rump, blade or eye fillet

2 teaspoons extra-virgin olive oil

2 teaspoons ground cumin

1 teaspoon sea salt flakes

12 metal skewers, or wooden skewers soaked in water

40 g (2 cups) baby spinach leaves

75 g (⅓ cup) Homemade Labne (page 222)

115 g (½ cup) Salsa Verde (page 227)

**GRILLED BROCCOLI**

1 tablespoon extra-virgin olive oil

1 head of broccoli, cut into quarters

Preheat the oven to 180°C.

Slice the steak into 5 mm pieces against the grain. Add to a bowl with the olive oil, cumin, salt and ¼ teaspoon freshly ground black pepper and toss to coat well. Thread the steak onto 12 skewers, then set aside.

Preheat a barbecue grill plate to high, or heat a cast-iron chargrill pan over high heat on the stovetop.

For the grilled broccoli, put the broccoli in a bowl, then add the olive oil and massage it into the broccoli pieces. Add the broccoli to the barbecue or chargrill pan and cook for 3 minutes on each side until charred. Transfer to a baking tray and cook in the oven for 20 minutes, until tender.

Keeping the barbecue or chargrill pan over high heat, add the steak skewers, cooking them for 3 minutes on one side, then flipping and cooking for another 1 minute (they should be charred but still pink through the middle). Set aside to rest until ready to serve.

Divide the steak skewers and grilled broccoli between four plates. Serve with the baby spinach and homemade labne and spoon some salsa verde over the top.

**Note** To turn this into an easy salad bowl, roughly chop the cooked broccoli and remove the grilled steak from the skewers. Toss in a bowl with the spinach, labne and salsa verde.

## BOOST

⌃ Roast 2 medium potatoes (300 g in total) with the broccoli to add to this meal. Extra 80 calories per serve.

 **SERVES** 4

 **PREP** 5 minutes

 **COOK** 30 minutes

 **CALS PER SERVE** 406

 **GLUTEN FREE**

 **ENTERTAINING**

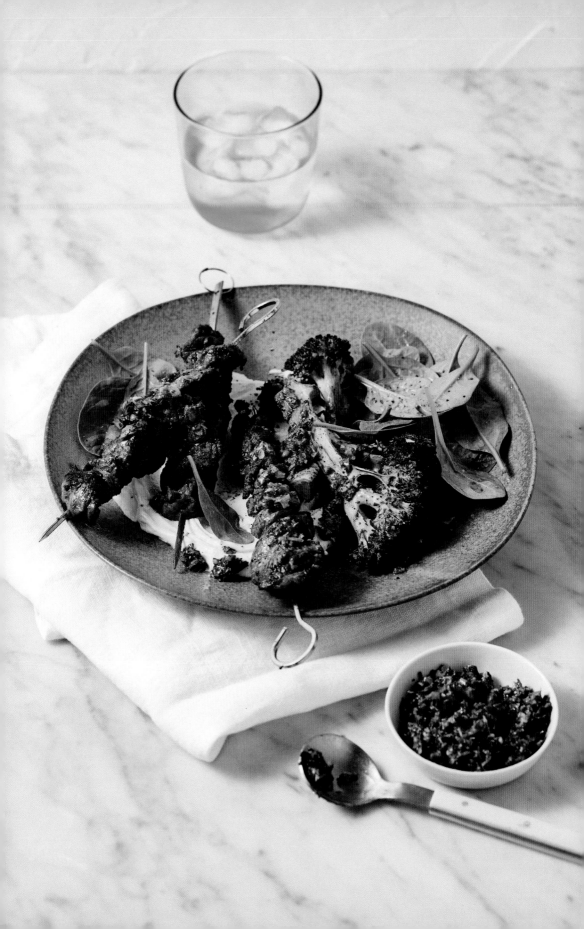

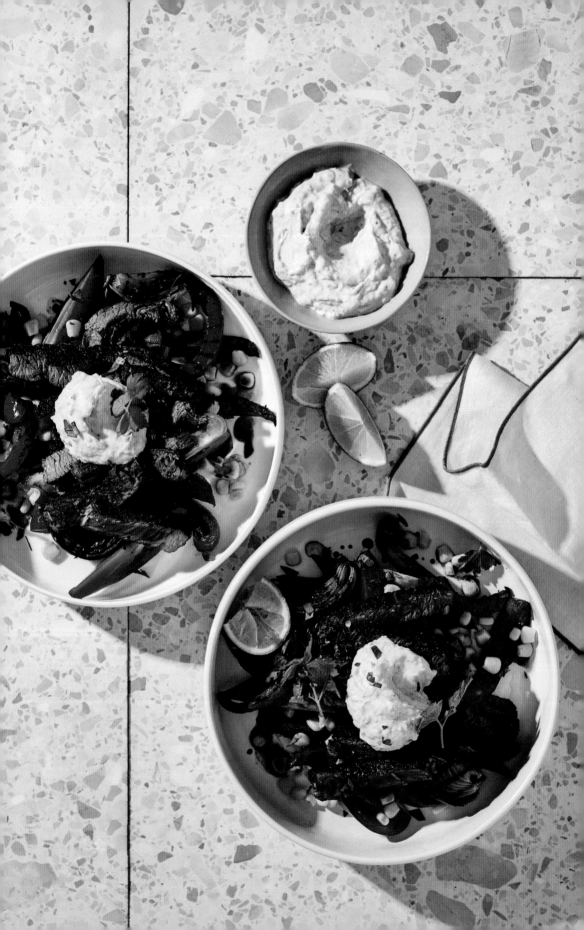

# BBQ Steak Fajita Bowl

Get ready to fiesta with this colourful, flavour-filled bowl of Mexican feasting! It's perfect for weeknights, great for leftovers and a delicious way to get your three veg in.

1 teaspoon extra-virgin olive oil

2 teaspoons dried oregano

2 teaspoons smoked paprika (see note)

½ teaspoon sea salt flakes

500 g lean beef steak, such as scotch fillet, rump, blade or eye fillet, trimmed of excess fat

1 red onion, cut into 1 cm slices

2 red capsicums, deseeded and cut into 1 cm slices

1 avocado

60 g (¼ cup) low-fat natural yoghurt

1 x 400 g can corn kernels, drained and rinsed

3 tomatoes, sliced

2 tablespoons finely chopped flat-leaf parsley

1 lime, sliced into wedges

Add the olive oil, oregano, paprika, salt and a pinch of freshly ground black pepper to a bowl and mix to combine. Massage this mixture into the steak on both sides.

Heat a barbecue grill plate to high, or heat a cast-iron chargrill pan over high heat on the stovetop. Once hot, add the steak and cook for 3 minutes on each side for medium–rare. Set aside and allow to rest for 10 minutes before cutting into 5 mm slices.

While the meat is resting, add the onion and capsicum to the hot barbecue or chargrill pan. Cook, tossing, for 5 minutes, until charred and tender.

Mash the avocado and yoghurt together with some salt and freshly ground black pepper.

Divide the grilled veggies and sliced steak between four bowls. Serve with the corn, tomato, parsley, avocado yoghurt and lime wedges.

**Note** You can replace the smoked paprika with 1 tablespoon store-bought Mexican spice blend.

## BOOST

☆ Serve each bowl with 2 x 25 g mini tortillas. Extra 156 calories per serve.

|  SERVES 4 |  PREP 10 minutes |  COOK 15 minutes |  CALS PER SERVE 393 |  GLUTEN FREE |  ENTERTAINING |

# Chargrilled Green Tomatoes & Lamb Chops with Pickled Yoghurt

Okay, if you haven't tried underripe green tomatoes, you must!
Tangy and firm (so they won't fall apart on the barbecue) they taste
A-MAZE-ZING with lemon, garlic and a little bit of chilli. Perfectly paired
with some lamb chops, chargrill the lot for a great summer night's feast!

2 teaspoons extra-virgin olive oil

12 lamb chops (1.3 kg), excess
   fat removed

2 cups rocket leaves

**GRILLED GREEN TOMATOES**

500 g green tomatoes, sliced
   1 cm thick

2 garlic cloves, minced

Juice of 1 lemon

¼ teaspoon dried chilli flakes

¼ teaspoon sea salt flakes

**PICKLE YOGHURT**

35 g (¼ cup) finely chopped
   gherkins

125 g (½ cup) low-fat natural
   yoghurt

To make the pickle yoghurt, add the gherkins and yoghurt to a bowl and mix to combine. Set aside.

Drizzle the olive oil over the lamb chops and season with salt and freshly ground black pepper. Massage the oil and seasoning into the meat.

For the grilled green tomatoes, put the tomatoes in a large bowl with the garlic. Sprinkle the lemon juice over and season with the chilli flakes, salt and a pinch of freshly ground black pepper. Toss to coat.

Preheat a barbecue grill plate to high, or heat a cast-iron chargrill pan over high heat on the stovetop, until it is almost smoking.

Add the tomatoes and lamb to the barbecue or chargrill pan. Cook the tomatoes for 2 minutes on each side until charred. Cook the lamb for 3 minutes on each side for medium. Transfer to a plate and allow to rest for a few minutes.

Divide the lamb chops, grilled green tomatoes, rocket leaves and the pickle yoghurt between four plates and serve.

**SERVES**
4

**PREP**
10 minutes

**COOK**
10 minutes

**CALS PER SERVE**
410

**GLUTEN FREE**

**20 MINUTES OR LESS**

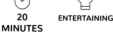
**ENTERTAINING**

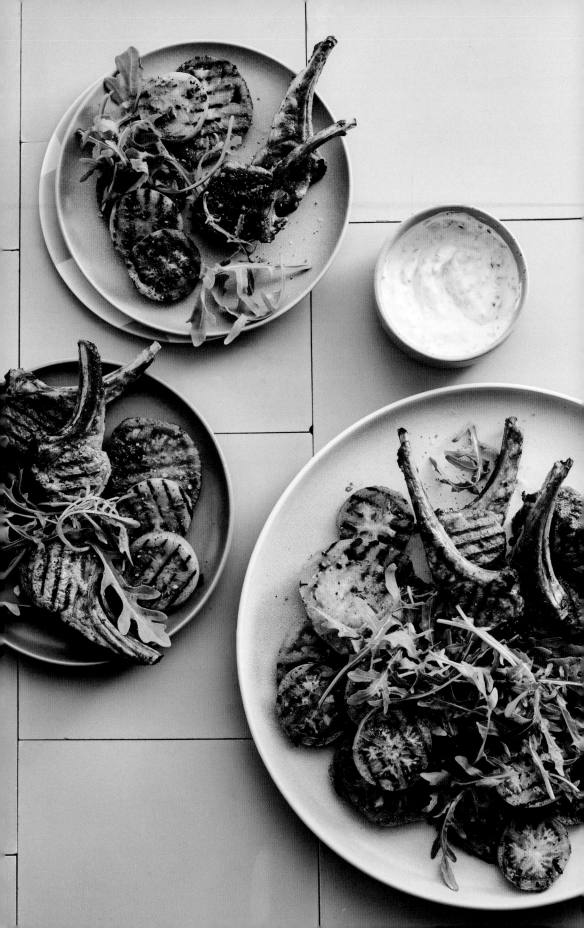

# Smoky Shredded Pork Tacos

Feasting on a fasting day? Can do! Perfect for dinner parties, this slow-roasted pork shoulder is so tender and juicy it falls off the bone. Enjoy with warm tortillas and crunchy fresh veg served with pickled onion.

550 g pork shoulder, trimmed of excess fat and cut into 3 cm chunks

2 teaspoons sea salt flakes

1 teaspoon extra-virgin olive oil

1 onion, finely diced

4 garlic cloves, minced

4 thyme sprigs, leaves picked

1 tablespoon ground cumin

1 tablespoon ground coriander

1 tablespoon apple cider vinegar

2 tablespoons chipotle chillies in adobo sauce

250 ml (1 cup) chicken stock

2 bay leaves

¼ green cabbage, finely sliced

1 cup coriander leaves

8 x 25 g mini flour or gluten-free tortillas, warmed

**QUICK PICKLED ONION**

¼ red onion, finely sliced

1 tablespoon red wine vinegar

Pinch of sea salt flakes

---

### BOOST

⌃ Serve each portion with 1 tablespoon of Salsa Verde (page 227 – extra 11 calories per serve) and ¼ small avocado (extra 30 calories per serve).

---

Preheat the oven to 180°C.

Season the pork with the salt and ¼ teaspoon freshly ground black pepper. Heat the olive oil in a large heavy-based ovenproof pot over medium–high heat. Once hot, add the pork and cook for 5 minutes, turning, until browned on most sides. Transfer to a bowl, leaving any residual fat in the pot.

Add the onion and garlic to the pot and cook for 3 minutes, until browned. Add the thyme, cumin and coriander and continue cooking for 1 minute. Pour the vinegar in and cook, stirring, for 30 seconds, scraping off any bits stuck to the bottom. Add the chillies, stock, bay leaves and pork. Stir, then bring to the boil. Remove from the heat, cover the pot with a lid, place in the oven and roast for 3 hours, until the pork is very tender. Remove the pot from the oven and lightly shred the pork using two forks. Place back in the oven, without the lid, and continue roasting for 30 minutes, until the water evaporates by half and the pork is crisp on the edges.

While the pork is in the oven, make the quick pickled onion by adding the ingredients to a small bowl and tossing to coat. Allow to sit until ready to serve.

Serve the shredded pork on a platter in the middle of the table with the pickled onion, sliced cabbage, coriander and warmed tortillas. Encourage guests to serve themselves.

**Note** Any extra shredded pork can be stored in an airtight container in the fridge for up to 5 days, or in the freezer for up to 3 months.

---

**SERVES**
4

**PREP**
10 minutes

**COOK**
3 hours
45 minutes

**CALS PER SERVE**
405

**GLUTEN FREE**

**ENTERTAINING**

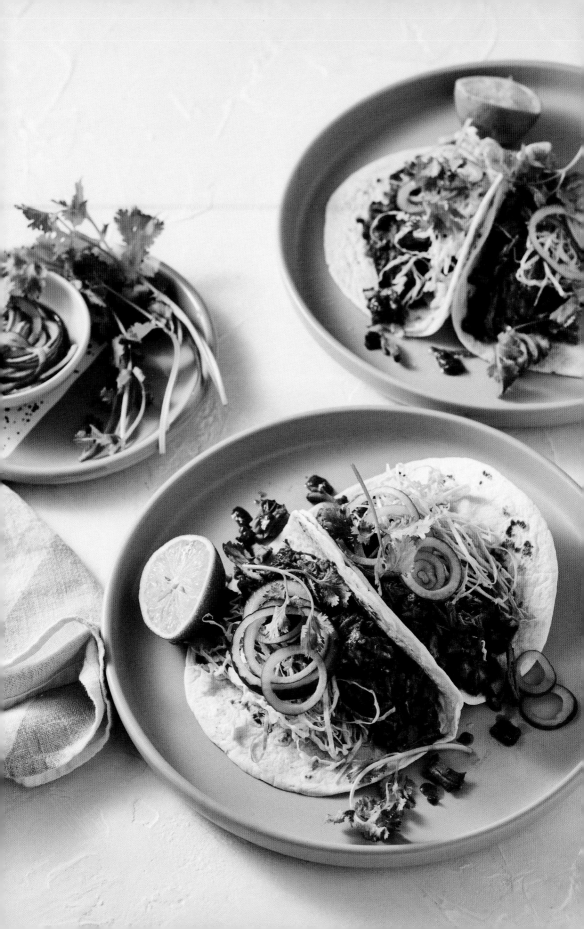

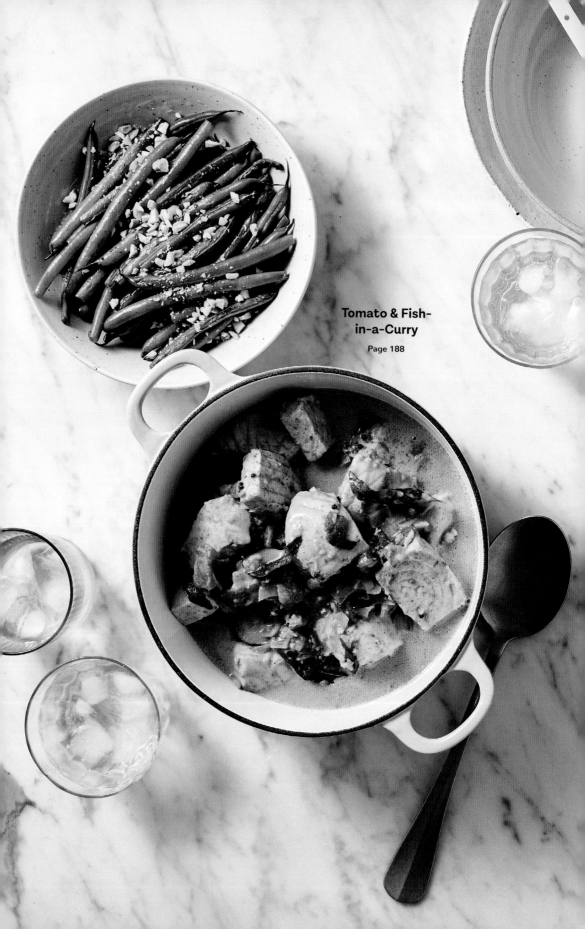

**Tomato & Fish-
in-a-Curry**

Page 188

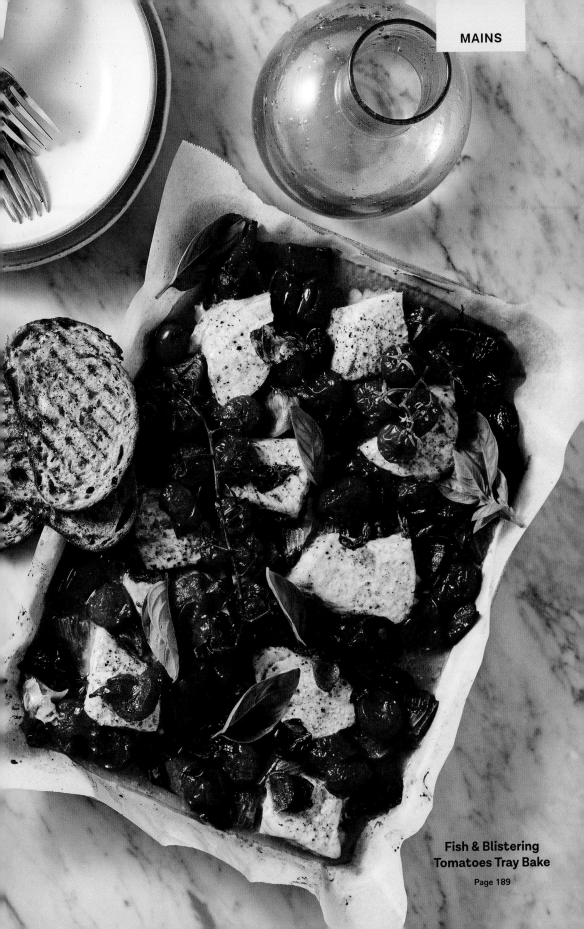

**Fish & Blistering
Tomatoes Tray Bake**

Page 189

# Tomato & Fish-in-a-Curry

This curry packs a flavour punch that's de-fish-iously intense! It'll be your new go-to recipe for rich, creamy curry without the calorie cost.

1 tablespoon extra-virgin
   olive oil
1 onion, finely diced
8 garlic cloves, minced
1 tablespoon finely minced
   ginger
200 g (1 cup) diced tomatoes
250 ml (1 cup) coconut milk
1 teaspoon sea salt flakes
600 g firm white fish (such as
   snapper or barramundi),
   cut into chunks
Juice of ½ lemon

**SPICE MIX (SEE NOTE)**

5 curry leaves
1 teaspoon ground turmeric
1 teaspoon brown mustard
   seeds
2 teaspoons ground coriander
1 teaspoon fennel seeds
1 teaspoon garam masala

**CHARRED GREEN BEANS**

2 teaspoons extra-virgin olive oil
300 g green beans, trimmed
1 tablespoon raw cashew nuts

Heat the olive oil in a large, deep, non-stick frying pan over medium heat. Once hot, add the onion and cook, tossing, for 3 minutes until browned. Add the garlic and ginger and continue to cook for 2 minutes, until golden and caramelised. Add the spice mix and cook, stirring, for 2 minutes until fragrant.

Add the tomatoes, coconut milk, salt and 250 ml (1 cup) water. Stir everything together and bring to a simmer. Add the fish pieces and continue cooking for 10–14 minutes, until the fish is just cooked through.

While the fish is cooking, make the charred green beans. Place the olive oil in a large frying pan over medium–high heat. Once hot, add the green beans and toss for 30 seconds to coat them in the oil. Cover the pan with a lid and cook, untouched, for 5 minutes, until lightly charred. Remove the lid, add the cashews and toss them through the beans. Continue to cook for another 2 minutes, until tender.

Divide the fish curry and charred green beans between four plates. Season with a little salt and freshly ground black pepper and serve.

## Notes

» You can swap the spice mix for 1½ tablespoons of a store-bought butter chicken or korma spice blend.
» To freeze, place portions of the curry in airtight containers and freeze for up to 3 months.

---
**BOOST**

⌃ Serve with 95 g (½ cup) of cooked basmati rice. Extra 100 calories per serve.

---

|  |  |  |  |   |  |
|---|---|---|---|---|---|
| **SERVES** 4 | **PREP** 10 minutes | **COOK** 25 minutes | **CALS PER SERVE** 400 | **GLUTEN FREE** | **DAIRY FREE** |

# Fish & Blistering Tomatoes Tray Bake

Seasonal tomatoes are so sensational they are bursting out of their skins in this rich, flavoursome fish dish! It comes together super easily and you'll be loving the delicious Mediterranean vibe of olives, capsicum, red onion, garlic and basil. Just close your eyes and dream of the Aegean ... happy sigh.

600 g cherry tomatoes

2 red capsciums, deseeded and chopped into 3 cm chunks

2 red onions, sliced 1 cm thick

10 kalamata olives, pitted and roughly chopped

4 garlic cloves, left in their skins

1 cup loosely packed basil leaves

1½ tablespoons extra-virgin olive oil

600 g white fish fillets (such as, snapper, barramundi, flathead), cut into even 10 cm pieces

4 slices (50 g each) sourdough bread, toasted

Pinch of sea salt flakes

Preheat the oven to 180°C.

Place the cherry tomatoes, capsicum, red onion, olives, garlic and basil across two large baking trays. Drizzle with the olive oil and toss to coat well. Bake in the oven for 25 minutes until the veggies are tender.

Remove from the oven, pick out the garlic and squeeze the flesh out of the skins back onto the baking tray. Using a fork, lightly crush the vegetables and mix them with the garlic, then place the fish fillets on top. Return to the oven for 10–12 minutes, until the fish is just cooked through.

Divide the fish, vegetables and toasted sourdough between four plates. Season with the salt and a pinch of freshly ground black pepper and serve.

**SERVES**
4

**PREP**
5 minutes

**COOK**
35 minutes

**CALS PER SERVE**
391

**DAIRY FREE**

# Chilli Prawn Omelette

Awesome fact 1: Eggs and prawns are packed full of protein. Awesome fact 2: They're also surprisingly low in calories! Best of all, protein is a satiating macronutrient, i.e. it keeps you fuller for longer. Here we add some delicious Asian flavours so you're not only eating smart – you're eating scrumptiously!

8 large free-range eggs

1 tablespoon fish sauce

500 g small cooked shelled and deveined prawns (see notes)

1 carrot, shredded

1 cup coriander, leaves picked, plus extra for serving

1 tablespoon sesame oil

75 g (½ cup) kimchi

1 tablespoon Chilli Sauce (page 227) or sriracha

45 g (⅓ cup) roasted, unsalted cashews, roughly chopped

Add the eggs and fish sauce to a medium bowl and whisk until well combined.

In another bowl, put the prawns, carrot and coriander and toss to combine.

Heat 1 teaspoon of the sesame oil in a medium non-stick frying pan over medium–high heat. Once hot, pour in one-quarter of the egg mixture and swirl to coat the base of the pan. Add one-quarter of the prawn mixture to one half of the pan. Cook for 1 minute, until the edges start to set, then flip the side of the omelette with no filling over the other half with the filling to enclose. Cook for a further minute, then remove from the pan and place on a plate. Repeat with the remaining egg and prawn mixture to make four omelettes in total.

Serve each chilli prawn omelette with kimchi and chilli sauce. Sprinkle with the roasted cashews and extra coriander leaves and serve.

## Notes

» If you're using frozen raw prawns, first thaw them in the fridge. Drain well. Heat a non-stick frying pan over medium heat. Add the raw prawns and toss for 3–4 minutes until they're cooked through – no oil needed! – then use as described in the recipe.

» Keep any left-over egg mixture in an airtight container or jar, and the prawn filling in an airtight container, for up to 3 days, so you can whip these omelettes up for a quick lunch.

**SERVES**
4

**PREP**
5 minutes

**COOK**
10 minutes

**CALS PER SERVE**
403

**GLUTEN FREE**

**DAIRY FREE**

**15 MINUTES OR LESS**

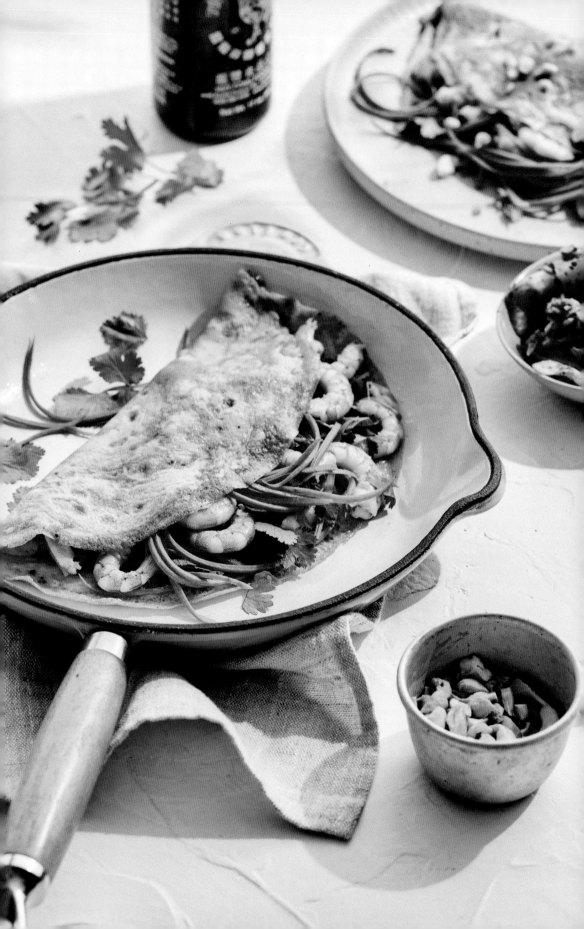

# Love This Jerk Salmon with Marinated Tomato Salsa

Huge on flavour, this Jamaican-inspired midweek dinner is ready in just 20 minutes so you can sit back, enjoy and dream of the Caribbean, baby.

600 g salmon fillets, skin on (4 x 150 g fillets)
1 teaspoon extra-virgin olive oil
200 g (1 cup) canned corn kernels, drained
2 x 45 g pita breads, cut in half, warmed

### MARINATED TOMATO SALSA

600 g cherry tomatoes, quartered
1 tablespoon finely chopped oregano (or ½ teaspoon dried oregano)
½ red onion, finely sliced
1 tablespoon red wine vinegar

### LEMONY LABNE

2 tablespoons Homemade Labne (page 222), or use store-bought
Juice of 1 lemon

### JERK SPICE BLEND

1 teaspoon dried thyme leaves
1 teaspoon ground allspice
1 teaspoon garlic powder
Pinch of cayenne pepper
Pinch of sea salt flakes
Pinch of freshly ground black pepper
1 teaspoon extra-virgin olive oil

Add all the ingredients for the marinated tomato salsa to a bowl. Mix to combine, then set aside to marinate while you prepare the rest of the meal.

For the lemony labne, add the homemade labne and lemon juice to a small bowl and mix to combine. Set aside.

Add all the ingredients for the jerk spice blend to a large shallow bowl and mix to combine. Put the salmon in the bowl and coat it with the spice mix on both sides.

Heat the olive oil in a large non-stick frying pan over medium–high heat. Once hot, add the salmon pieces, skin-side down. Cook for 5 minutes until the skin is crispy, then flip and continue cooking for another 3–4 minutes until the fish is cooked to your liking. Transfer to a plate to rest.

Drain out any excess oil from the pan, leaving just a little in the bottom. Place back over medium–high heat and add the corn kernels. Cook, tossing for 3 minutes, until tender.

Divide the jerk salmon, corn, marinated tomato salsa and pita halves between four plates. Drizzle with the lemony labne, season with a generous amount of freshly ground black pepper and a little salt and serve.

### BOOST

⌃ Add an additional 2 x 45 g small pita breads, so each serve has 1 whole pita.
Extra 124 calories per serve.

**SERVES**
4

**PREP**
5 minutes

**COOK**
15 minutes

**CALS PER SERVE**
400

**20 MINUTES OR LESS**

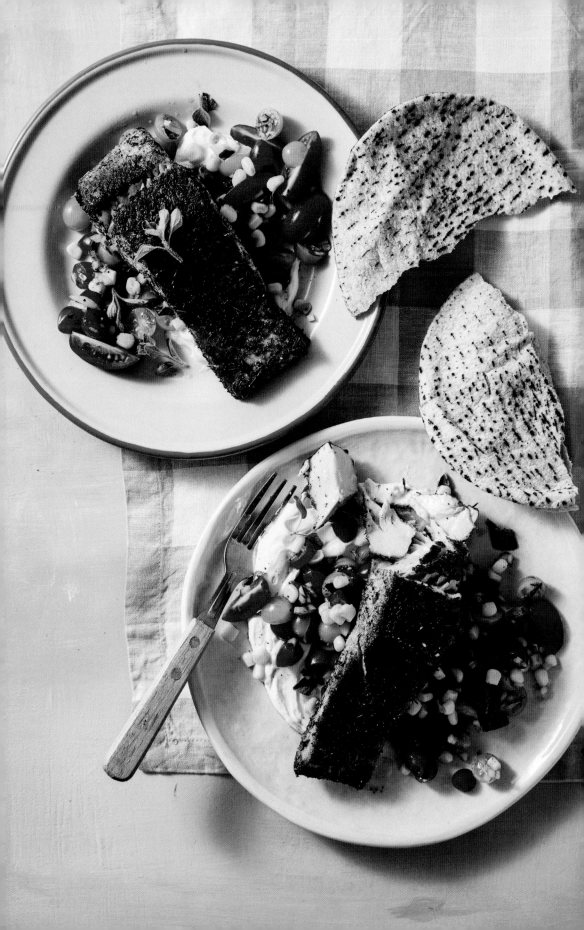

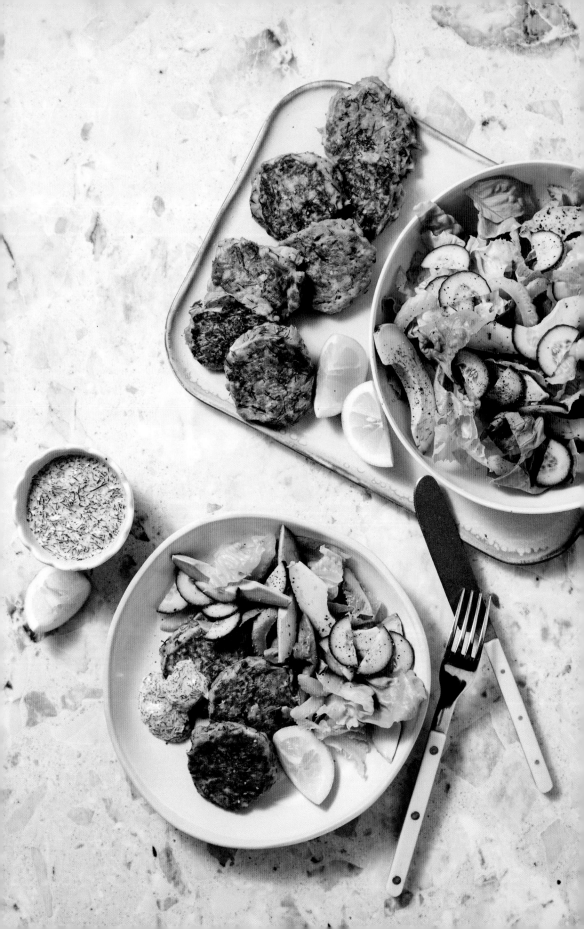

# Tasty Fishcakes with Cucumber Salad & Creamy Dressing

We should really call this creamy dressing 'dreamy dressing' because it's so divine! And these easy, crispy fishcakes are just made to pair with the dressing. We've used canned salmon in spring water, which is both a cost-effective and super easy way to get some healthy, oily fish into your diet. Serve with cucumber salad and you've got summer on a plate.

**SALMON FISHCAKES**

500 g drained tinned salmon in spring water (about 800 g before draining)
2 x large free-range eggs
2 spring onions, finely sliced
¼ cup dill leaves, finely chopped, plus extra to serve
Zest of 1 lemon
35 g (¼ cup) plain flour
1 tablespoon dijon mustard
1 tablespoon extra-virgin olive oil

**CREAMY DRESSING (SEE NOTES)**

85 g (⅓ cup) mayonnaise
1 teaspoon dijon mustard
Juice of ½ lemon
1 bunch of dill, finely chopped
¼ teaspoon sea salt flakes
¼ teaspoon freshly ground black pepper

**CUCUMBER SALAD**

4 cups roughly torn butter lettuce
2 Lebanese cucumbers, finely sliced
2 celery stalks, finely sliced
1 small avocado, sliced

To make the fishcakes, add the salmon to a large mixing bowl and use the back of a fork to mash and flake the salmon. Add the eggs, spring onion, dill and lemon zest. Mix well, then add the flour and fold it through. Use a ¼ cup measure to scoop up 12 portions of the batter and form into patties.

Heat a drizzle of the olive oil in a large frying pan over medium heat. Add the fishcakes, four at a time, cooking for 4 minutes on each side, until golden brown on the exterior and the egg has set. Set aside and repeat with the remaining mixture.

To make the creamy dressing, add all the ingredients to a small bowl and mix well to combine.

To make the cucumber salad, add all of the ingredients to a large bowl and toss to combine. Divide the fishcakes and cucumber salad between four bowls.

Spoon some creamy dressing over the top, garnish with the extra dill, season with freshly ground black pepper and serve.

## Notes

» Instead of the creamy dressing, you can just serve each portion with 1 tablespoon of mayonnaise.
» To freeze, individually wrap each uncooked fishcake in baking paper and place in an airtight container. Freeze for up to 3 months.

**SERVES**
4

**PREP**
20 minutes

**COOK**
20 minutes

**CALS PER SERVE**
378

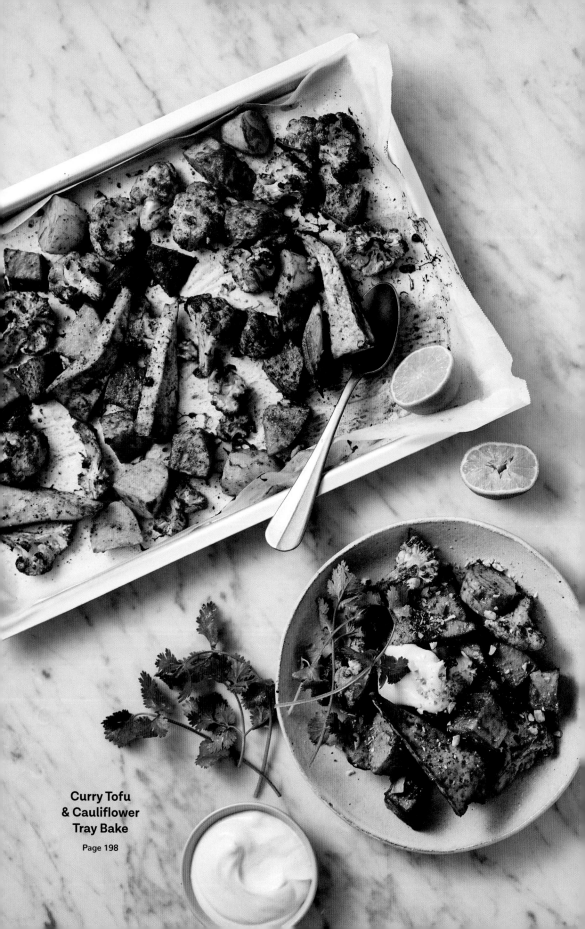

**Curry Tofu
& Cauliflower
Tray Bake**

Page 198

Sumac Chickpeas
& Tomato Salad
Pita Chip Crunch

Page 199

# Curry Tofu & Cauliflower Tray Bake

Curry is king in our kitchens, but getting out the whole spice cabinet and laboriously grinding them all in a mortar and pestle thingy is definitely in the too-hard basket. Enter one of our fave hacks: curry paste! You can make a delicious meal without the fuss AND this dinner allows for less cleaning up too! #lifestooshortforkitchenslaving

125 g (½ cup) low-fat natural yoghurt
1 tablespoon yellow curry paste
500 g potatoes, roughly chopped into 2 cm pieces
1 small head (450 g) cauliflower, florets and stems cut into 2 cm pieces
300 g pumpkin, peeled and chopped into 2 cm pieces
1 red onion, sliced into 1 cm thick wedges
350 g firm tofu, sliced into 2 cm triangles

**TO SERVE**
130 g (½ cup) low-fat natural yoghurt
40 g (¼ cup) Salsa Verde (page 227) or 1 cup roughly chopped coriander leaves
50 g (⅓ cup) unsalted, roasted cashews nuts, roughly chopped
1 lime, sliced into wedges

Preheat the oven to 180°C.

Place the yoghurt and curry paste in a large bowl and mix to combine. Add the potato, cauliflower, pumpkin, red onion and tofu and toss gently to coat everything in the curried yoghurt.

Spread the mixture across two large baking trays and place in the oven. Roast for 30 minutes, until everything is golden on the edges and the veggies are tender when pierced with a knife.

Divide the curry-roasted vegetables and tofu between four bowls. Dollop the yoghurt on top and sprinkle with the salsa verde and cashews. Serve with lime wedges.

**SERVES**
4

**PREP**
10 minutes

**COOK**
30 minutes

**CALS PER SERVE**
399

**GLUTEN FREE**

**VEGETARIAN**

# Sumac Chickpeas & Tomato Salad Pita Chip Crunch

A super simple, meat-free Monday recipe that only takes 20 minutes to make? Yes please! Better still, make a double batch of these delish sumac chickpeas for protein-rich snacky munchies and salad sensation crunchies later in the week.

2 large pita breads, sliced into 3 cm pieces
2 x 400 g cans chickpeas, drained and rinsed
1 tablespoon sumac
3 teaspoons extra-virgin olive oil
600 g cherry tomatoes, halved
2 Lebanese cucumbers, sliced
½ red onion, finely sliced
1 tablespoon red wine vinegar
½ teaspoon sea salt flakes
1 cup flat-leaf parsley, finely chopped
½ cup dill sprigs, finely chopped
4 tablespoons (4 serves) Roasted Garlic Cream (page 220) or low-fat natural Greek yoghurt
1½ tablespoons roughly chopped roasted almonds

Preheat the oven to 180°C.

Spread the pita pieces across a large baking tray.

Place the chickpeas on another large baking tray and sprinkle with the sumac and olive oil and toss to coat.

Place both trays in the oven and bake for 10 minutes until the pita and chickpeas are golden brown.

Meanwhile, place the cherry tomatoes, cucumber, red onion, red wine vinegar, salt, parsley and dill in a large bowl and toss to combine.

Divide the tomato salad, pita chips and sumac chickpeas between four bowls. Spoon the roasted garlic cream over the top, scatter with the almonds and serve.

Note To make this vegan, use coconut yoghurt in place of the roasted garlic cream or Greek yoghurt.

**SERVES**
4

**PREP**
10 minutes

**COOK**
10 minutes

**CALS PER SERVE**
398

**VEGETARIAN**

**20 MINUTES OR LESS**

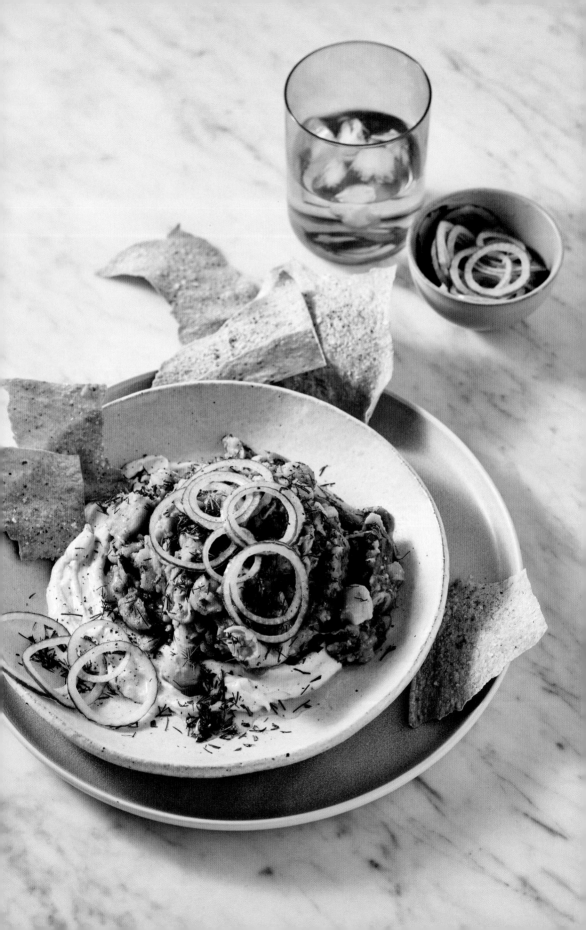

# Smoky BBQ Eggplant with Butter Beans

Chargrilled eggplant and creamy butter beans make for one delicious meat-free meal! The tahini garlic yoghurt is bound to become a favourite – it's perfect with anything on the grill or tossed through a noodle salad.

3 eggplants (1 kg in total)

1 teaspoon sea salt flakes

Juice of 1 lemon

1½ tablespoons extra-virgin olive oil

2 x 440 g cans butter beans, drained and rinsed

125 g (½ cup) Roasted Garlic Cream (page 220) or low-fat natural yoghurt

2 tablespoons tahini

½ red onion, finely sliced

1 cup roughly chopped flat-leaf parsley

½ cup roughly chopped dill leaves

4 x 25 g mountain bread wraps, to serve (toasted if you like, see notes)

Preheat a barbecue grill to high. Prick the eggplants all over with a fork, then place them on the barbecue and cook, for 25 minutes, turning occasionally, until the skin is blackened and charred. Place in a large bowl, cover with foil and allow the eggplants to steam and cool down for 10 minutes.

Peel the skin from the eggplant and discard, then roughly chop the flesh. Place in a bowl and toss with the salt, lemon juice and 1 tablespoon of the olive oil. Add the butter beans and toss them through, crushing them gently with a spoon. (Taste the eggplant at this stage – see if you'd like to add any more salt or lemon, as it soaks up this flavour!)

Combine the roasted garlic cream and tahini in a bowl.

Divide the barbecued eggplant and the butter beans between four bowls. Generously top with the onion slices and herbs. Drizzle with the remaining 2 teaspoons of olive oil and serve each bowl with mountain bread wraps to tear and scoop up the mixture.

## Notes

» To toast mountain bread wraps, preheat the oven to 180°C. Roughly tear the mountain bread into large pieces and place across baking trays. Bake in the oven for 10 minutes until golden brown around the edges.

» You can also cook the eggplants on a gas stovetop over medium heat. Place the eggplant directly on the open flame. Cook for 15 minutes, turning every few minutes, until the skin is blackened and charcoal. Place in a bowl and cover with foil to steam and cool down for 10 minutes. Continue with the recipe.

**SERVES**
4

**PREP**
20 minutes

**COOK**
25 minutes

**CALS PER SERVE**
399

**VEGETARIAN**

# Tofu Ramen Bowl of Goodness

This nourishing vegan bowl is like a big, warm hug and is packed full of protein and flavour. There's also a high water content to keep you hydrated and fuller for longer. Get ready to bowl over those calorie goals!

3 teaspoons extra-virgin olive oil

500 g firm tofu, chopped into 2 cm cubes

600 g mushrooms (Swiss brown, shiitake, oyster etc.)

4 garlic cloves, finely sliced

2 teaspoons miso paste

1 tablespoon tahini

60 ml (¼ cup) tamari or soy sauce

2 teaspoons vegetable stock powder

180 g dried ramen noodles

2 zucchini, shredded into long thin strips like spaghetti, or spiralised

2 cups shredded kale

4 spring onions, finely chopped

Heat half the olive oil in a large heavy-based saucepan over medium–high heat. Once hot, add the tofu and cook, tossing, for 5 minutes until golden brown on all sides. Remove the tofu from the pan and set aside. Add the remaining oil and mushrooms and cook, stirring, for 3 minutes until browned and tender. Add the garlic and stir it through for 1 minute, until fragrant.

Add 1.5 litres of water to the pan, along with the miso paste, tahini, tamari or soy sauce, stock powder and noodles. Bring to the boil, then reduce to a simmer and cook for 3–4 minutes, until the ramen noodles are tender (or cook for as long as the packet instructions say).

Add the zucchini, kale and reserved tofu to the pan and stir for 1 minute until the kale is wilted, the zucchini is just tender and the tofu is warmed through. Divide the ramen between four serving bowls and garnish with the spring onion.

## BOOST

≽ Add 1 medium boiled egg for a more traditional way to serve ramen. Extra 60 calories per serve.

**SERVES**
4

**PREP**
10 minutes

**COOK**
25 minutes

**CALS PER SERVE**
396

**DAIRY FREE**

**VEGAN**

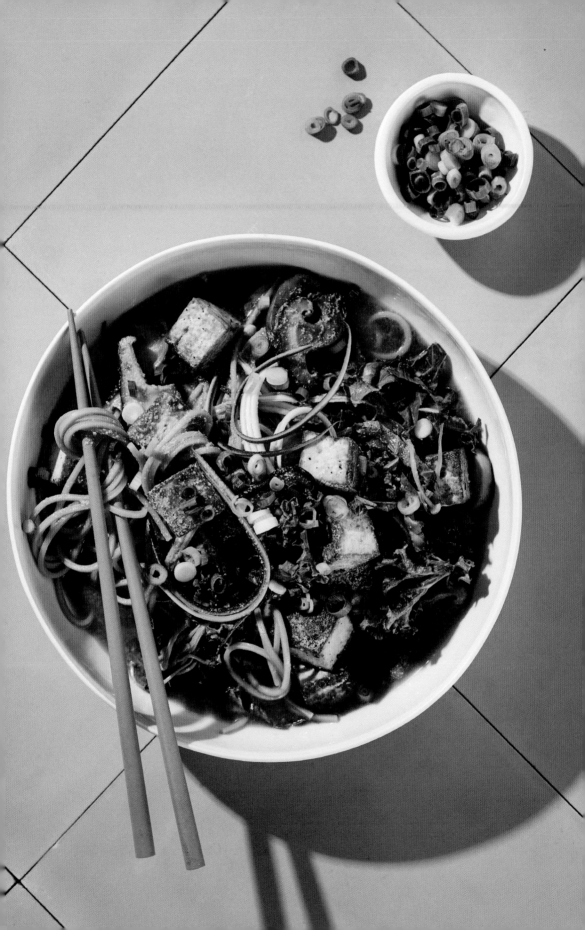

# Roasted Broccoli & White Bean Comfort Soup

Nothing nourishes like a warm, cheesy bowl of delicious and hearty soup. Make a double batch and freeze portions so, on those days when you say there's 'nothing to eat', it's comfort soup to the rescue!

3 heads broccoli, florets and stems roughly chopped into 3 cm pieces
1 onion, sliced 1 cm thick
8 garlic cloves, left in their skins
1 tablespoon extra-virgin olive oil
1 litre (4 cups) vegetable or chicken stock
2 x 400 g cans white beans, drained and rinsed (yields about 3 cups)
Juice of 1 lemon
30 g shaved parmesan
4 slices wholemeal bread, toasted

Preheat the oven to 180°C.

Spread the broccoli, onion and garlic across two large baking trays. Drizzle with the olive oil and season generously with salt and freshly ground black pepper. Toss to coat, then bake in the oven for 20–25 minutes, until the veggies are browned and the broccoli florets are charred.

Remove the veggies from the oven and place the broccoli and onion in a medium saucepan (reserving some roasted broccoli for garnish, if you like). Squeeze the garlic flesh out of the skins into the pan, then add the stock and white beans. Use a stick blender to blitz the soup until smooth. Heat over medium–high heat and bring to a simmer. Cook for 2–3 minutes, until warmed through. Turn off the heat, and stir through the lemon juice.

Divide the soup between four bowls and top with the reserved roasted broccoli and shaved parmesan. Garnish with a little more freshly ground black pepper and serve with the toast.

**Note** Divide the soup into individual portions and freeze for up to 3 months.

**SERVES**
4

**PREP**
10 minutes

**COOK**
25 minutes

**CALS PER SERVE**
398

**VEGETARIAN**

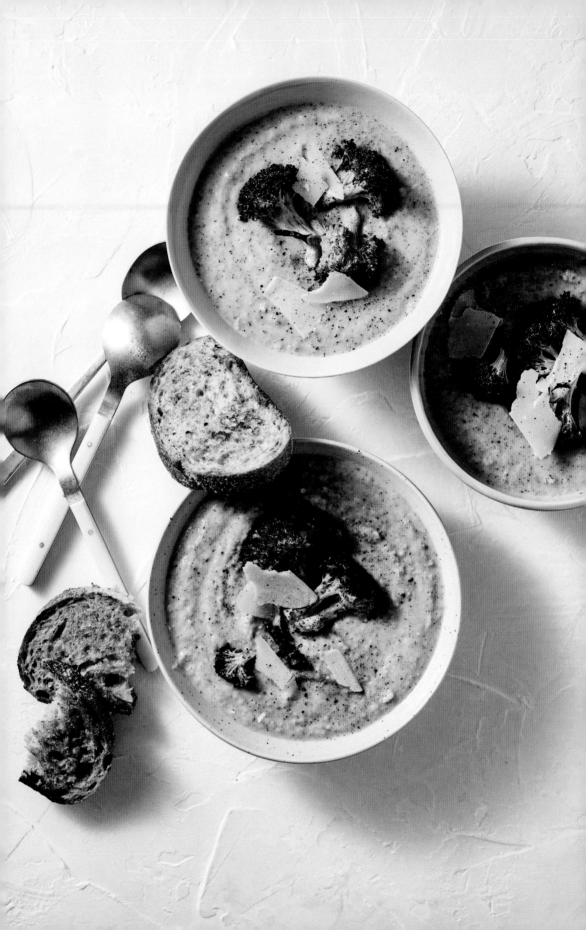

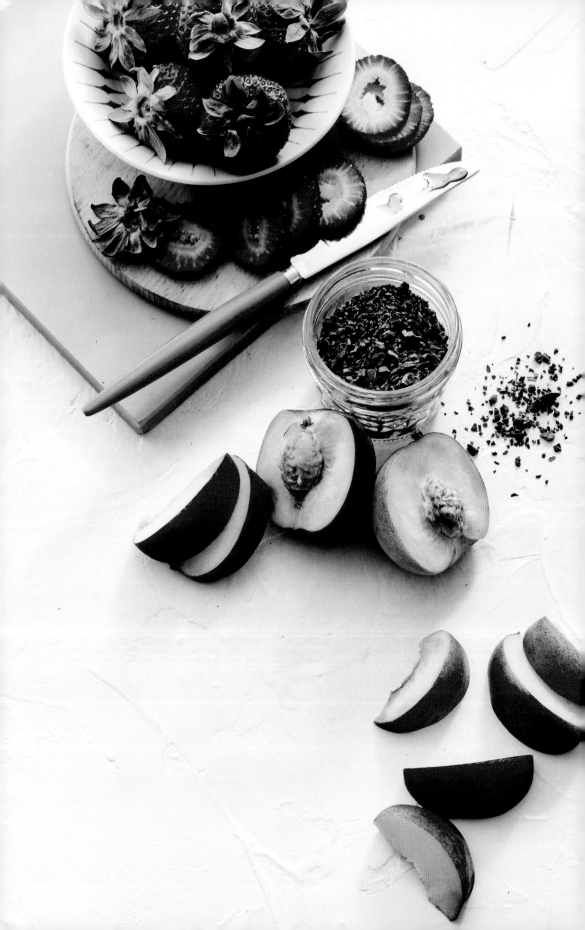

# Snacks & treats

Who doesn't love a good snack? And it's even better when you can munch away without blowing your cals. Each and every one of these recipes is a tried and tested favourite of ours and has helped us drop kilos easily without ever feeling like we're missing out, especially if we're having a cuppa or a cheeky glass of wine. #sfdlife

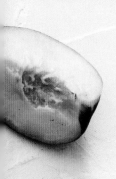

# Cucumber Cream Cheese Sandwiches

What to eat when hunger strikes? Try these super low-cal snacks! Fresh cucumber and cream cheese is already a winner, but when topped with our Everything Bagel Seasoning it becomes extra scrummy.

2 Lebanese cucumbers, sliced 5 mm thick

125 g (½ cup) low-fat cream cheese

2 tablespoons Everything Bagel Seasoning – make your own (see below) or use store-bought

**EVERYTHING BAGEL SEASONING**

2 teaspoons white sesame seeds

2 teaspoons black sesame seeds

1¼ teaspoons dried onion flakes

1¼ teaspoons dried garlic flakes

1 teaspoon sea salt flakes

½ teaspoon poppy seeds

If making your own bagel seasoning, add all the seasoning ingredients to a jar and shake to combine.

Lay half the cucumber slices flat and spread the cream cheese between them. Sprinkle with the bagel seasoning, then top with the other half of the cucumber slices. Divide between four plates and serve.

**SERVES**
4

**PREP**
5 minutes

**CALS PER SERVE**
93

**GLUTEN FREE**

**VEGETARIAN**

**5 MINUTES OR LESS**

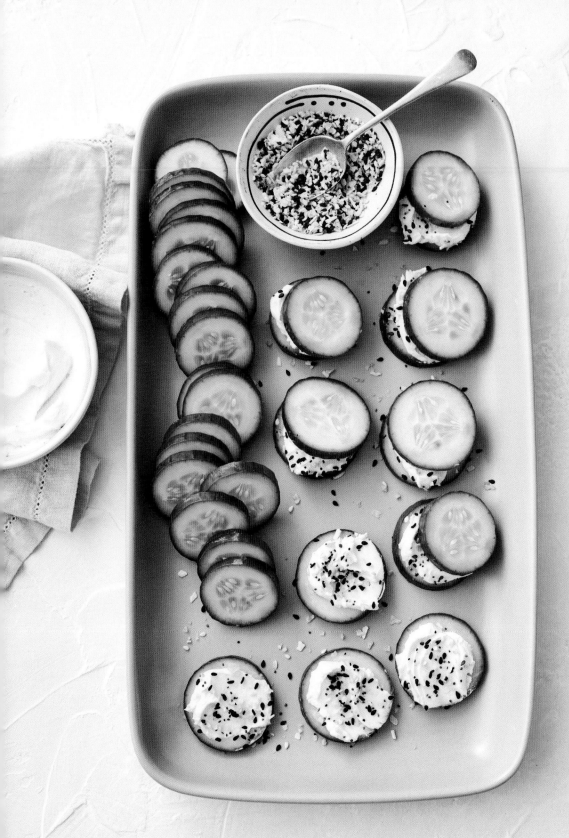

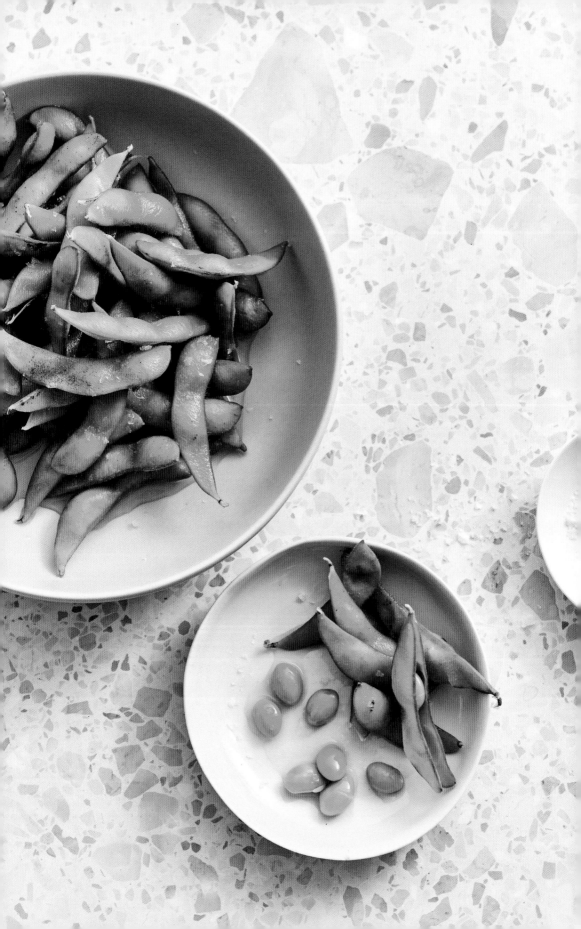

# Salt & Vinegar Edamame

Ahh, edamame ... what a craving saver you are! Keeping bags of frozen edamame on hand is a great idea, as you can simply boil some water and dump them in at any time. Edamame is the perfect snack as it's high in protein and fibre – the ideal combo to help keep you satiated until your next meal. This recipe works a treat because you're also getting your salt and vinegar fix, without the high cals.

2 teaspoons cooking salt
250 g frozen edamame pods
2 teaspoons rice wine vinegar
1 teaspoon sea salt flakes

Fill a medium saucepan with water, add the cooking salt and bring to the boil. Add the frozen edamame and cook according to the packet instructions.

Drain, then add to a serving bowl. Drizzle with the vinegar and toss to coat. Sprinkle with the sea salt and serve.

**SERVES**
4

**PREP**
2 minutes

**COOK**
10 minutes

**CALS PER SERVE**
100

**GLUTEN FREE**

**DAIRY FREE**

**VEGAN**

**10 MINUTES OR LESS**

# Oaty Peach Crumble

Butter, cinnamon, juicy peaches ... what's not to love about this food-comfort crumble? Fibre-rich peaches are a healthy, sweet treat, but you can use any fruit in season. Strawberries, blueberries or apples would all work well, making this a recipe for all year round.

4 peaches, stones removed, chopped into 2 cm dice
1 tablespoon cornflour or tapioca flour
½ teaspoon ground cinnamon
2 teaspoons honey

**CRUMBLE TOPPING**
100 g (1 cup) rolled quick oats
2 tablespoons apple sauce

Preheat the oven to 180°C and lightly spray a small 20 cm baking dish with oil.

Place the chopped peaches, cornflour and cinnamon in the baking dish and toss to coat the peaches well. Drizzle with the honey and toss again to coat. Add 1-4 tablespoons of water to the peaches, until they're well lubricated and juicy (this will depend on how ripe your peaches are!).

For the crumble topping, add the oats to a bowl with the apple sauce. Use your fingers to combine the ingredients until the mixture holds together in clumps. Sprinkle this mixture over the peaches.

Bake the crumble in the oven for 30–40 minutes, until it is bubbling around the edges and the top is golden brown.

Divide between six small bowls to serve.

---

**BOOST**

☆ Serve with 1 tablespoon of low-fat natural yoghurt
Extra 11 calories per serve.

---

 **SERVES** 6

 **PREP** 10 minutes

 **COOK** 30 minutes

 **CALS PER SERVE** 103

 **DAIRY FREE**

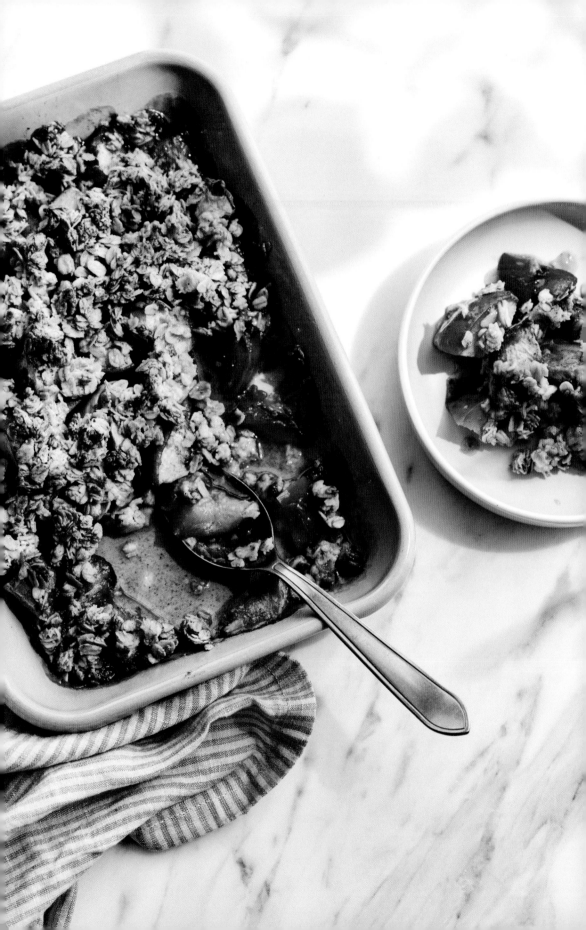

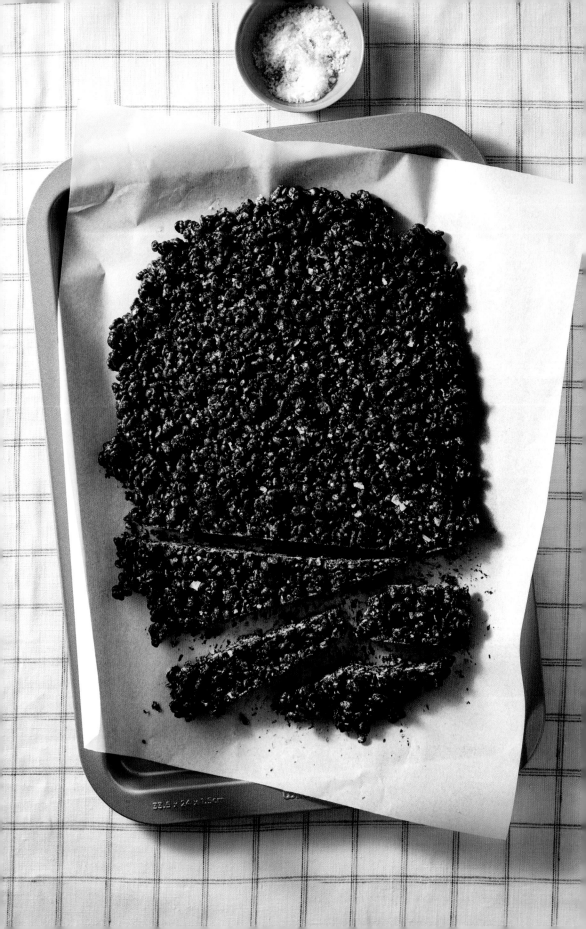

# Chocolate Crackle Bites

When chocolate cravings strike, you'll be stoked to have a batch of these super yummy chocolate crackle bites in the freezer. We've used tahini here for a rich, sesame flavour, but you can swap it out for a nut butter of your choice. It's crackling good stuff!

---

85 g dark chocolate (70% cocoa), roughly chopped
2 tablespoons tahini
90 g (3 cups) puffed rice
Pinch of sea salt flakes

Line a baking tray with baking paper.

Add the dark chocolate and tahini to a medium saucepan over medium–low heat. Heat, stirring, for 4 minutes, until completely melted and combined. Remove from the heat, add the puffed rice and stir it through until completely covered in the chocolate mixture.

Transfer the mixture to the baking tray and flatten it out, pushing down on the mixture with the base of a cup, until smooth. Sprinkle with a little salt, then place in the freezer for 30 minutes, or until set.

Slice into shards to serve.

**Note** Store the frozen chocolate crackle bites in an airtight container or ziplock bag in the freezer for up to 3 months.

---

## BOOST

⌃ Add 35 g (¼ cup) of chopped macadamias to the mixture. Extra 30 calories per serve.

---

**SERVES**
8

**PREP**
2 minutes + 1 hour setting time

**COOK**
5 minutes

**CALS PER SERVE**
101

**GLUTEN FREE**

# Strawberry Coco Froyo

Craving ice-cream? We so get that! But there is an alternative that's lower in calories and still heavenly! Go coco froyo – a blend of frozen strawberries with luscious coconut yoghurt that we cream to create a thick and dreamy after-dinner treat.

420 g (3 cups) frozen strawberries
2 teaspoons honey
125 g (½ cup) coconut yoghurt, frozen into ice-cubes
60 g (¼ cup) coconut yoghurt
1 teaspoon natural vanilla extract
1 tablespoon flaked coconut (optional)

Add all the ingredients, except the flaked coconut, to a food processor or high-powered blender. Pulse until the ingredients become smooth. Add 60–125 ml (¼–½ cup) of water to allow the ingredients to blend smoothly. It will take 2–5 minutes to blend the mixture, so keep going! You want this mixture to be a nice and thick ice-cream consistency!

Divide between four little cups and top with the coconut to serve.

**Note** You can store the froyo in the freezer in an airtight container for up to 3 months. To serve, allow to thaw for 3–5 minutes to soften slightly before eating. Or try freezing this froyo in popsicle moulds.

 **SERVES** 4

 **PREP** 10 minutes

 **CALS PER SERVE** 99

 **GLUTEN FREE**

**DAIRY FREE**

 **10 MINUTES OR LESS**

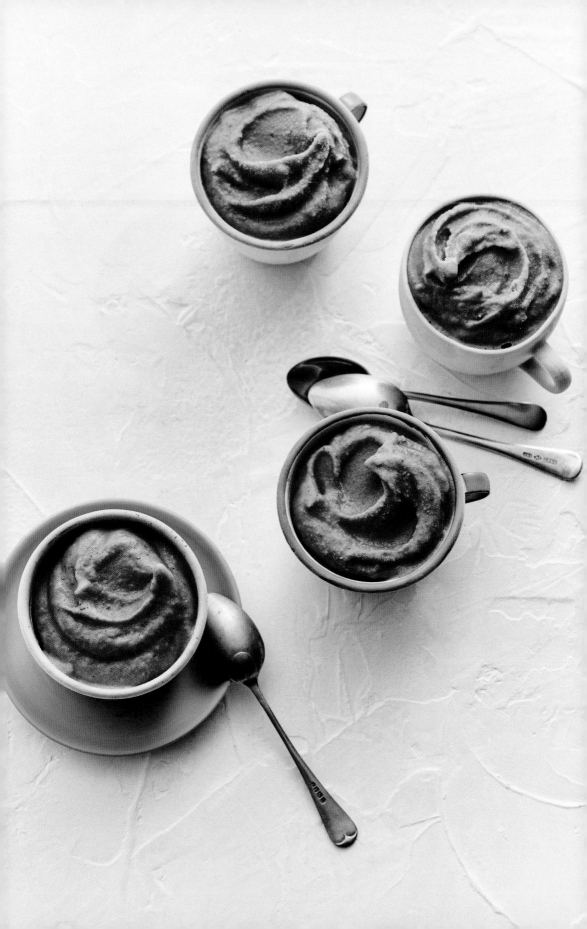

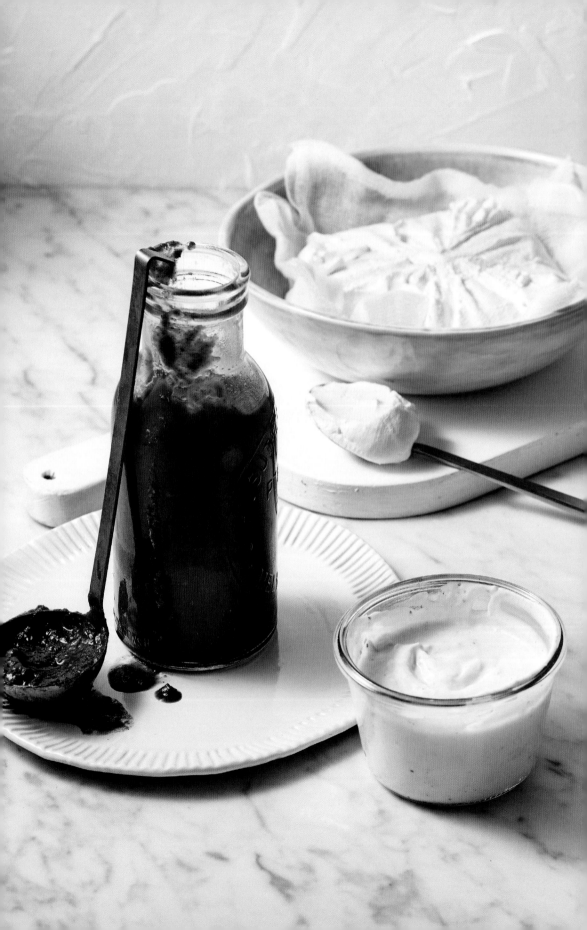

# Basics

Well, we say basics but these recipes are actually luxury extras that you will absolutely love adding to your meals and snacks. Sometimes a little creamy, spicy, smoky goodness can go a long, delicious way.

# Roasted Garlic Cream

This is the perfect accompaniment to all your chargrilled proteins and salads – or is great just served on crackers as a snack. Sometimes it's the little things that can make the whole meal.

1 garlic bulb
250 g (1 cup) low-fat natural
    yoghurt
Juice of ½ lemon
½ teaspoon sea salt flakes

Preheat the oven to 180°C.

Separate the garlic cloves, leaving their skins on. Place the cloves on a baking tray, then roast for 20 minutes, until the garlic is squishy when squeezed with tongs.

Remove the roasted garlic from the oven and allow to cool for 2 minutes. Squeeze the garlic from its skins into a bowl. Mash the garlic with a fork, then add the yoghurt, lemon juice, salt and ¼ teaspoon freshly ground black pepper. Mix well until combined.

Place in an airtight container or jar. The cream will last for 5 days in the fridge.

**MAKES**
250 g (1 cup) 12 serves,
1 tablespoon per serve

**PREP**
5 minutes

**COOK**
20 minutes

**CALS PER SERVE**
12

**GLUTEN FREE**

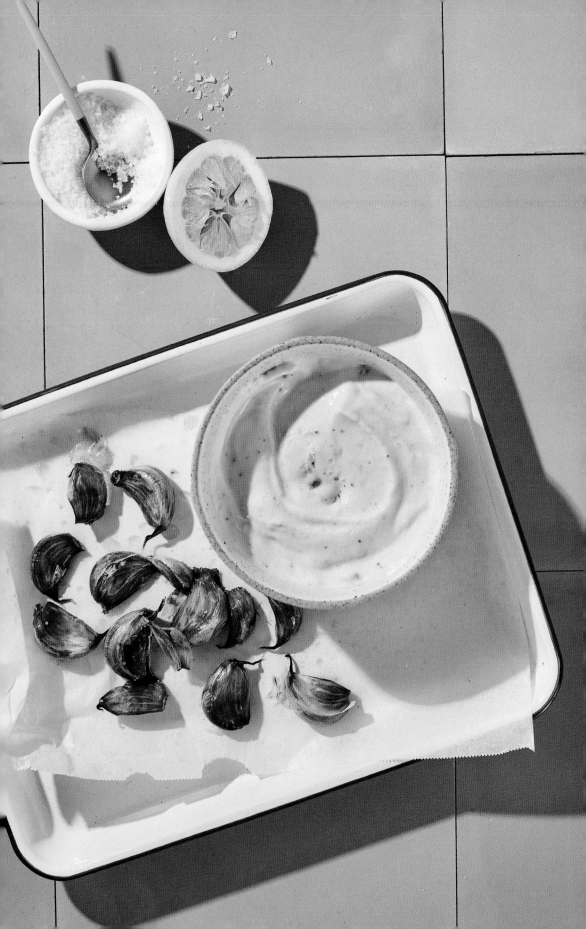

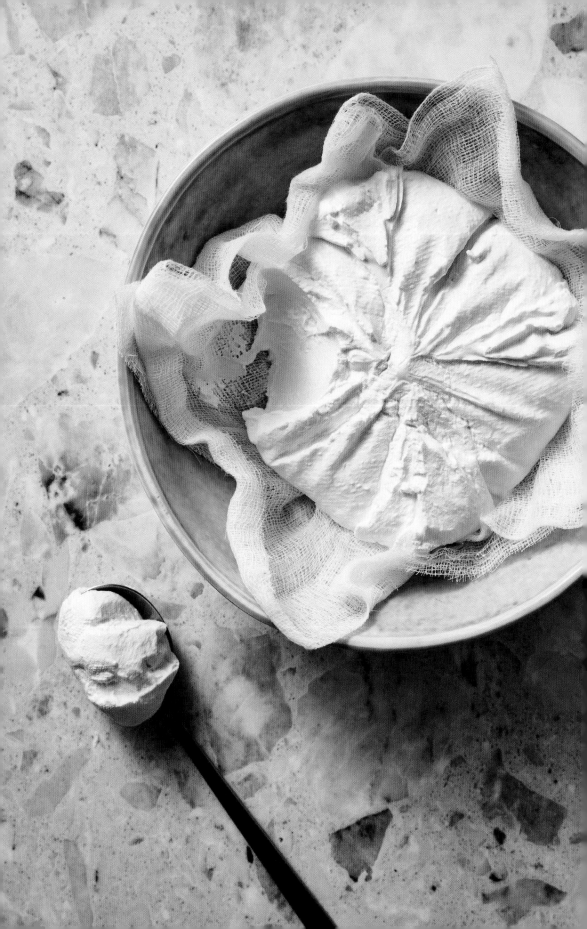

# Homemade Labne

Labne is an extremely delicious, creamy condiment to eat with dips and dressings or to serve alongside protein, but you'll pay an exorbitant price if you buy it. This homemade recipe is super easy and will save you money – plus it's totally yum. Enjoy!

500 g (2 cups) full-fat Greek
    yoghurt
½ teaspoon sea salt flakes
Cheesecloth (or porous kitchen
    cloth, like Chux)

Combine the yoghurt and salt in a bowl.

Place a layer of cheesecloth over a large bowl and scoop the yoghurt into the middle of the cloth. Tie the cheesecloth together in a knot, then place the bundle in a sieve set over the bowl. Place a tea towel over the top of the bowl.

Leave on the kitchen bench for 24 hours. After this time the yoghurt will separate into solids (the labne) and drip the liquid (whey) into the bowl. Discard the whey and transfer the labne to an airtight container. The labne is now ready to use.

**Note** Store the labne in an airtight container in the fridge for up to 1 week.

**MAKES**
225 g (1 cup) serves 12,
1 tablespoon per serve

**PREP**
4 minutes,
plus setting

**CALS PER
SERVE**
47

**GLUTEN
FREE**

# Smoky BBQ Sauce

A sugar-free, low-calorie barbecue sauce that's super rich and tasty – and with a calorie count so low you can slather it to your heart's content.

450 g (2½ cups) tomato passata
1 tablespoon tamari
  or soy sauce
60 ml (¼ cup) water
125 ml (½ cup) apple cider
  vinegar
1 tablespoon honey
1 tablespoon dijon mustard
1 teaspoon onion powder
1 teaspoon garlic powder
2 teaspoons smoked paprika
½ teaspoon freshly ground
  black pepper
½ teaspoon salt

Heat all the ingredients in a medium saucepan over medium heat until you reach a slow boil. Reduce the heat to low and simmer for 15–20 minutes until the sauce is thick and a deep red colour. Remove from the heat and allow to cool before transferring into an airtight container or jar.

The sauce will keep in the fridge for up to 1 week.

**Note** You can freeze the sauce in a standard ice cube tray. Once frozen, pop out the cubes and store in an airtight container or ziplock bag in the freezer for up to 3 months.

**MAKES**
600 g (2 cups) 24 serves,
1 tablespoon per serve

**PREP**
5 minutes

**COOK**
25 minutes

**CALS PER
SERVE**
11

**GLUTEN
FREE**

**DAIRY
FREE**

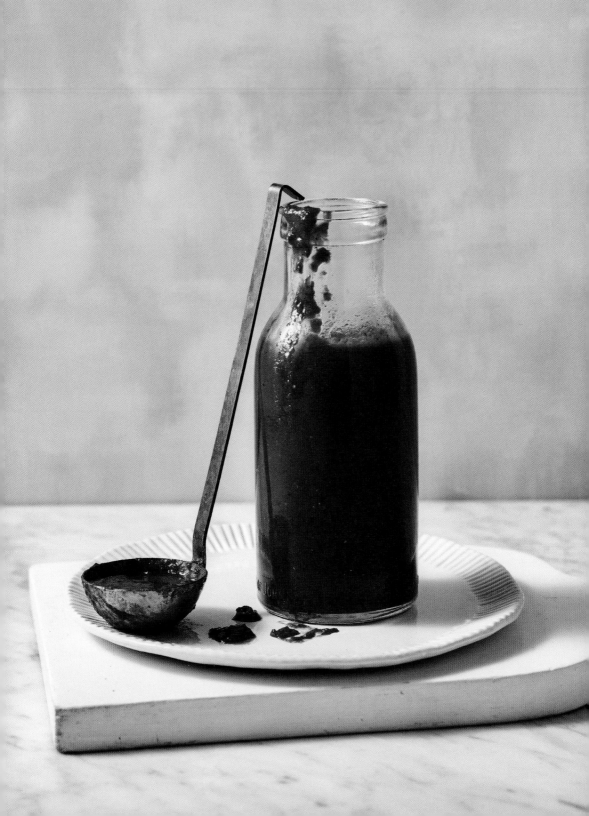

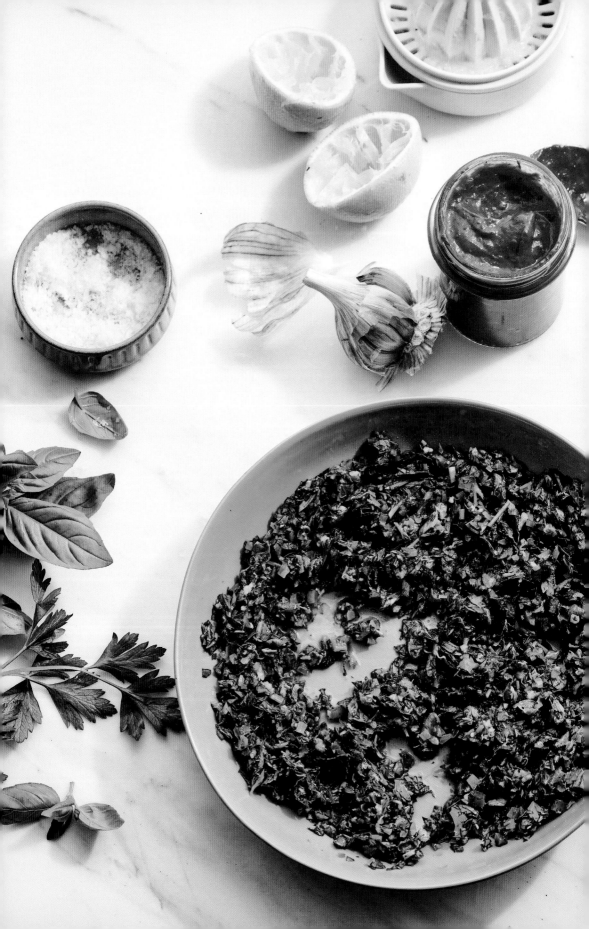

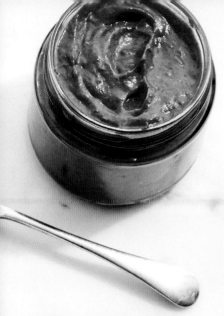

# Hot Chilli Sauce

We're claiming it – this is the best homemade hot chilli sauce EVER! We recommend making a double (or triple) batch and storing it in the fridge for a few weeks to allow the flavours to settle and develop. It won't go to waste – we promise.

Makes: 500 g (2½ cups) 120 serves, 1 teaspoon per serve
Prep time: 10 minutes • Cooking time: 25 minutes
Calories per serve: 3 • Gluten-free • Dairy-free

1 garlic bulb
4–6 long red chillies
3 red capsicums, deseeded and roughly chopped
2 golden shallots, peeled (sweet onions)
1 tablespoon extra-virgin olive oil
¼ teaspoon sea salt flakes
60 ml (¼ cup) apple cider vinegar

Preheat the oven to 180°C.

Separate the garlic cloves, leaving their skins on. Place the garlic, chillies, capsicum and shallots on a baking tray. Drizzle with the olive oil and season with the salt and ¼ teaspoon freshly ground black pepper and toss to coat. Bake for 25 minutes until everything is softened and lightly charred.

Remove from the oven and allow to cool slightly before transferring the chilli, capsicum and shallots into a food processor. Squeeze the garlic out of its skin and into the food processor, add the apple cider vinegar and blitz to a chunky paste. Add 375 ml (1½ cups) of water and blitz again to thin out the sauce.

Transfer the hot chilli sauce into a jar or bottle and store in the fridge until needed. The sauce will continue to develop in flavour over time (it's best 2–3 weeks after you make it!) and will last up to 6 months in the fridge.

# Salsa Verde

Yum, yum, yum! This go-to condiment is the perfect accompaniment to steak, chicken or tofu plus you can toss it through salads, spread it on toast or serve it with fried eggs. Salsa verde traditionally contains olive oil, but we've made this version without it, keeping it so low-calorie that you can salsa away, every day!

Makes: 340 g (1⅓ cups) 8 serves, 2 tablespoons per serve
Prep time: 20 minutes • Calories per serve: 11
Gluten-free • Dairy-free

1 bunch of flat-leaf parsley, finely chopped
1 bunch of basil, leaves picked and finely chopped
2 tablespoons capers in vinegar, finely chopped
2 tablespoons finely chopped gherkins
2 garlic cloves, minced
1 teaspoon dijon mustard
Juice of 1 lemon
2 teaspoons red wine vinegar
1 teaspoon sea salt flakes
½ teaspoon chilli flakes
½ teaspoon freshly ground black pepper

Put all the ingredients in a bowl. Stir together until well combined, then allow to sit for 30 minutes for the flavours to come together and release some more liquid.

Place in an airtight container or jar and keep for 3–5 days in the fridge.

# Endnotes

## Chapter 1

P 22 The latest data from the Australian Bureau of Statistics (ABS) ... Australian Bureau of Statistics, *Overweight and obesity*, December 2018, www.abs.gov.au

P 24 Fasting also increases 'good' cholesterol ... Falek Zeb et al., 'Effect of time-restricted feeding on metabolic risk and circadian rhythm associated with gut microbiome in healthy males', *The British journal of nutrition*, vol. 123, no. 11, 2020, p. 1216–26.

P 24 A 2020 study on the effects of fasting ... Hyueyun Kim et al., 'The Impact of Time-Restricted Diet on Sleep + Metabolism in Obese Volunteers', *Medicina*, vol. 56, no. 10, 2020, p. 540.

P 24 Multiple studies found a reduction in waist circumference ... Emily N C Manoogian et al., 'Time-restricted Eating for the Prevention and Management of Metabolic Diseases', *Endocrine reviews*, vol. 43, no. 2, 2022, p. 405–426.

P 24 One study reporting a median decrease ... Malini Prasad et al., 'A Smartphone Intervention to Promote Time Restricted Eating Reduces Body Weight and Blood Pressure in Adults with Overweight and Obesity: A Pilot Study', *Nutrients*, vol. 13, no. 7, 2021, p. 2148.

P 24 It may help prevent cancer ... Tatiana Moro et al., 'Time-restricted eating effects on performance, immune function, and body composition in elite cyclists: a randomized controlled trial', *Journal of the International Society of Sports Nutrition*, vol. 17, no. 1, 2020, p. 65.

P 24 In 2020, a study found that in excess, IGF-1 ...: Anika Knuppel et al., 'Circulating Insulin-like Growth Factor-I Concentrations and Risk of 30 Cancers: Prospective Analyses in UK Biobank', *Cancer research*, vol. 80, no. 18, 2020, p. 4014–21.

P 25 It may improve quality of life ... Katharina Anic et al., 'Intermittent Fasting—Short- and Long-Term Quality of Life, Fatigue, and Safety in Healthy Volunteers: A Prospective, Clinical Trial', *Nutrients*, vol. 14, 2022, p. 4216.

P 25 It may increase energy ... Katharina Anic et al., 'Intermittent Fasting—Short- and Long-Term Quality of Life, Fatigue, and Safety in Healthy Volunteers: A Prospective, Clinical Trial', *Nutrients*, vol. 14, 2022, p. 4216.

P 25 It may improve brain function ... Mark P Mattson & Ruiqian Wan, 'Beneficial effects of intermittent fasting and caloric restriction on the cardiovascular and cerebrovascular systems', *The Journal of nutritional biochemistry*, vol. 16, no. 3, p. 129–137.

P 25 It may decrease blood pressure ... Krista A Varady et al., 'Cardiometabolic Benefits of Intermittent Fasting', *Annual review of nutrition*, vol. 41, 2021, p. 333–361.

P 25 A review of studies that looked at the mental health effects ... Elisa Berthelot et al., 'Fasting Interventions for Stress, Anxiety and Depressive Symptoms: A Systematic Review and Meta-Analysis', *Nutrients*, vol. 13, no. 11, 2021, p. 3947.

## Chapter 2

P 34 Fasting allows our bodies to run ... Satchin Panda, *The Circadian Code*, Penguin Random House, London, 2018, p. 192.

P 34 A healthy fat cell can be 90% fat ... Satchin Panda *The Circadian Code*, Penguin Random House, London, 2018, p. 200.

P 41 There are some genetic factors that mean some people .... J A Levine, N L Eberhardt & M D Jensen, 'Role of nonexercise activity thermogenesis in resistance to fat gain in humans', *Science*, vol. 283, no. 5399, 1999, p. 212–14.

P 42 A review of scientific studies that examined ... Katherine Sievert et al., 'Effect of breakfast on weight and energy intake: systematic review and meta-analysis of randomised controlled trials', *British Medical Journal*, vol. 364, 2019, p. 142.

P 43 In our review of studies that tested the effects of fasting on sleep ... Mara McStay et al., 'Intermittent Fasting and Sleep: A Review of Human Trials', *Nutrients*, vol.13, no. 10, p. 3489.

## Chapter 3

P 52 However, research suggests that waiting 60 minutes ... Emily N C Manoogian et al., 'Time-restricted Eating for the Prevention and Management of Metabolic Diseases', *Endocrine reviews*, vol. 43, no. 2, 2022, p. 405–436.

P 52 This is partly because our bodies ... Emily N C Manoogian, Amandine Chaix & Satchidananda Panda, 'When to Eat: The Importance of Eating Patterns in Health and Disease. Journal of biological rhythms', vol. 34, no. 6, 2019, p. 579–81.

P 57 In general, a weight loss goal that's between ... Krista A Varady et al., 'Cardiometabolic Benefits of Intermittent Fasting', *Annual review of nutrition*, vol. 41, 2021, p. 333–61.

## Chapter 4

**P 70 One study compared the effect of processed food ...**
Kevin D Hall et al., 'Ultra-Processed Diets Cause Excess
Calorie Intake and Weight Gain: An Inpatient Randomized
Controlled Trial of Ad Libitum Food Intake', *Cell
metabolism*, vol. 30, no. 1, 2019, p. 67–77.

**P 70 In 2022, the Australian Bureau of Statistics reported**
... Australian Bureau of Statistics, *Dietary behaviour*, June
2022, www.abs.gov.au

**P 71 Fruits and vegetables are loaded** ...National
Health and Medical Research Council, *Australian Dietary
Guidelines*, 2013, www.eatforhealth.gov.au

**P 73 It told the brain-bridge on you** ... B Benelam,
'Satiation, satiety and their effects on eating behaviour',
*Nutrition Bulletin*, vol. 34, no. 2, 2009, p. 126–73.

**P 73 This may sound counter-productive** ... Kevin D Hall
et al., 'Energy balance and its components: implications for
body weight regulation', *The American journal of clinical
nutrition*, vol. 95, no. 4, 2012, p. 989–94.

**Top Ten Real Food Superstars** ... Nutritional content from
Harvard School of Public Health, *The Nutrition Source*,
2022, www.hsph.harvard.edu/nutritionsource/; caloric
content from www.fatsecret.com.au

**P 79 This can vary depending on the amount of fibre** ...
Kevin D Hall et al., 'Energy balance and its components:
implications for body weight regulation', *The American
journal of clinical nutrition*, vol. 95, no. 4, 2012, p. 954–94.

**P 82 According to the latest ABS statistics** ... *Australian
Bureau of Statistics, Australian Health Survey: Usual
Nutrient Intakes*, March 2015, www.abs.gov.au

**P 82 In Australia, sucrose (a simple sugar extracted
from sugar cane)** ...National Health and Medical
Research Council, *Australian Dietary Guidelines*, 2013,
www.eatforhealth.gov.au

## Chapter 5

**P 88 Studies show that people tend to consume** ...
B Benelam, 'Satiation, satiety and their effects on eating
behaviour', *Nutrition Bulletin*, vol. 34, no. 2, 2009,
p. 126–73.

**P 90 The National Health and Medical Research Council
of Australia suggests** ... National Health and Medical
Research Council, *Australian guidelines to reduce health
risks from drinking alcohol*, 2020, www.nhmrc.gov.au

**P 96 Studies also show that ghrelin tends** ... Mari
Näätänen et al., 'Post-weight loss changes in fasting
appetite- and energy balance-related hormone
concentrations and the effect of the macronutrient content
of a weight maintenance diet: a randomised controlled
trial', *European Journal of Nutrition*, vol. 60, 2021,
p. 2603–16.

**P 96 Interestingly, research shows that people with
obesity** ... M D Klok, S Jakobsdotti & M L Drent, 'The role
of leptin and ghrelin in the regulation of food intake and
body weight in humans: a review', *Obesity Reviews*, vol. 8,
no. 1, 2007, p. 21–34

**P 96 One study compared the appetites** ... Pauline
Oustric et al., 'Food Liking but Not Wanting Decreases
after Controlled Intermittent or Continuous Energy
Restriction to ≥5% Weight Loss in Women with
Overweight/Obesity', *Nutrients*, vol. 13, no. 1, 2021,
p. 182.

**P 97 Unfortunately, less than 25% of people** ...Australian
Bureau of Statistics. *Physical activity*, March 2022,
www.abs.gov.au

**P 98 A 2022 study found that a light walk** ... Aidan J
Buffey et al., 'The Acute Effects of Interrupting Prolonged
Sitting Time in Adults with Standing and Light-Intensity
Walking on Biomarkers of Cardiometabolic Health in
Adults: A Systematic Review and Meta-analysis', *Sports
Medicine* vol. 52, no. 8, 2022, p. 1765–87.

**P 98 Almost 50% of Australians report** ... Australian
Institute of Health and Welfare, *Sleep problems as
a risk factor for chronic conditions*, November 2021,
www.aihw.gov.au

**P 98 Scientists have found an association between
short sleep** ... Jianfei Lin et al., 'Associations of short
sleep duration with appetite-regulating hormones and
adipokines: A systematic review and meta-analysis',
*Obesity Reviews*, vol. 21, no. 11, 2020, p. 13051.

**P 98 Another study in overweight adults** ... Esra Tasali
et al., 'Effect of Sleep Extension on Objectively Assessed
Energy Intake Among Adults With Overweight in Real-
life Settings: A Randomized Clinical Trial', *Journal of the
American Medical Association Internal Medicine*, vol. 182,
no. 4, 2022, p. 365–74.

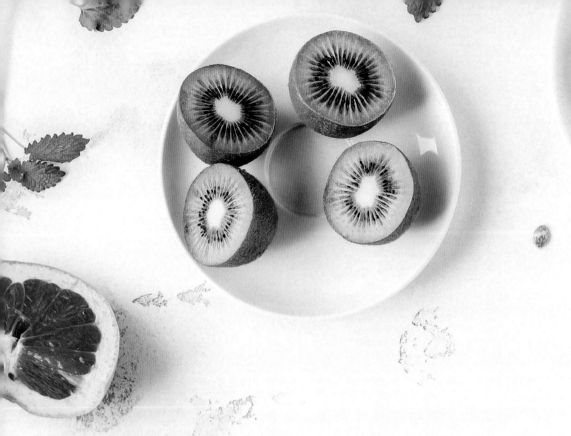

# Thank you! Thank you! Thank you! 🙏

We cannot begin to express how grateful we are to everyone who gave their heart and soul to this brilliant book of transformation. 🤍🖤💚

Firstly, to our terrific team at SuperFastDiet . . .

Our word magician and chief researcher, Alegria Alano – you are a scientific genius and fabulous storyteller.

Our food goddess, Meg Yonson – your creativity and enthusiasm for creating to-die-for dishes is highly contagious!

Maryanne O'Connor, your word-polishing and cheeky jokes are delightful.

Nicola Daniels, our General Manager. You are our rock! There's no way we could do what we do without you.

Kirsten Wenborne, for the sensational meal plans and nutritional wisdom.

Kimberlee Kessler, our Brand Champion – you are the head of making things beautiful.

Thanks also to our incredible team, especially Vanessa Giblin, Jacki Smith, Kristin McDonnell, Emily Ogden, Joyce Lonzaga and Luiza Amaral, plus Angie O'Reilly, Joanna Benson and all our amazing Super Coaches.

Not to mention a gigantic, super-duper thank you to all our case studies and SuperFastDiet.com members for inspiring us every day with your enthusiasm and awesome transformations.

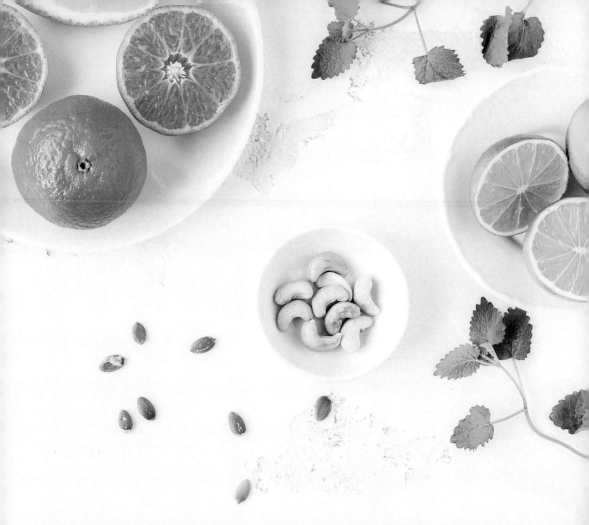

Thanks a million also to the phenomenal Dr Jason Fung and Megan Ramos for generously sharing their latest research and clinical findings on the incredible benefits of intermittent fasting with us. Thanks to Dr Krista's PhD students and postdoctoral fellows for running all these intermittent fasting clinical trials. You are the best.

All the Pan Macmillan stars who have made creating this book a complete joy, led by the super-professional, clever and gorgeous publisher Ingrid Ohlsson – thank you for your unwavering faith in us and this awesome way of life. And to the phenomenal PM team: Ariane Durkin, Lucinda Thompson, Sally Devenish and Jane Watkins. Big thanks also to designer Madeleine Kane, editor Ariana Klepac, photographers Rob Palmer and Jeremy Simons, food stylists Vanessa Austin and Emma Knowles and prep chef Kerrie Ray.

And a special thanks to our families:
Victoria: John, Myles, Bryce and Lloyd
Gen: Paul and Juliette
Krista: Nicolas, Gabriel, Jacob, Lou, and Eva.

Thank you so very much for all your love and support.

You are all our superheroes!
Biggest love,

Vic, Gen and
Dr. Krista xx

# Conversion chart

Measuring cups and spoons may vary slightly from one country to another, but the difference is generally not enough to affect a recipe. All cup and spoon measures are level. One Australian metric measuring cup holds 250 ml (8 fl oz), one Australian metric tablespoon holds 20 ml (4 teaspoons) and one Australian metric teaspoon holds 5 ml. North America, New Zealand and the UK use a 15 ml (3-teaspoon) tablespoon.

## Length

| METRIC | IMPERIAL |
| --- | --- |
| 3 mm | ⅛ inch |
| 6 mm | ¼ inch |
| 1 cm | ½ inch |
| 2.5 cm | 1 inch |
| 5 cm | 2 inches |
| 18 cm | 7 inches |
| 20 cm | 8 inches |
| 23 cm | 9 inches |
| 25 cm | 10 inches |
| 30 cm | 12 inches |

## Liquid measures

| ONE AMERICAN PINT | ONE IMPERIAL PINT |
| --- | --- |
| 500 ml (16 fl oz) | 600 ml (20 fl oz) |

| CUP | METRIC | IMPERIAL |
| --- | --- | --- |
| ⅛ cup | 30 ml | 1 fl oz |
| ¼ cup | 60 ml | 2 fl oz |
| ⅓ cup | 80 ml | 2½ fl oz |
| ½ cup | 125 ml | 4 fl oz |
| ⅔ cup | 160 ml | 5 fl oz |
| ¾ cup | 180 ml | 6 fl oz |
| 1 cup | 250 ml | 8 fl oz |
| 2 cups | 500 ml | 16 fl oz |
| 2¼ cups | 560 ml | 20 fl oz |
| 4 cups | 1 litre | 32 fl oz |

## Dry measures

The most accurate way to measure dry ingredients is to weigh them. However, if using a cup, add the ingredient loosely to the cup and level with a knife; don't compact the ingredient unless the recipe requests 'firmly packed'.

| METRIC | IMPERIAL |
| --- | --- |
| 15 g | ½ oz |
| 30 g | 1 oz |
| 60 g | 2 oz |
| 125 g | 4 oz (¼ lb) |
| 185 g | 6 oz |
| 250 g | 8 oz (½ lb) |
| 375 g | 12 oz (¾ lb) |
| 500 g | 16 oz (1 lb) |
| 1 kg | 32 oz (2 lb) |

## Oven temperatures

| CELSIUS | FAHRENHEIT |
| --- | --- |
| 100°C | 200°F |
| 120°C | 250°F |
| 150°C | 300°F |
| 160°C | 325°F |
| 180°C | 350°F |
| 200°C | 400°F |
| 220°C | 425°F |

| CELSIUS | GAS MARK |
| --- | --- |
| 110°C | ¼ |
| 130°C | ½ |
| 140°C | 1 |
| 150°C | 2 |
| 170°C | 3 |
| 180°C | 4 |
| 190°C | 5 |
| 200°C | 6 |
| 220°C | 7 |
| 230°C | 8 |
| 240°C | 9 |
| 250°C | 10 |

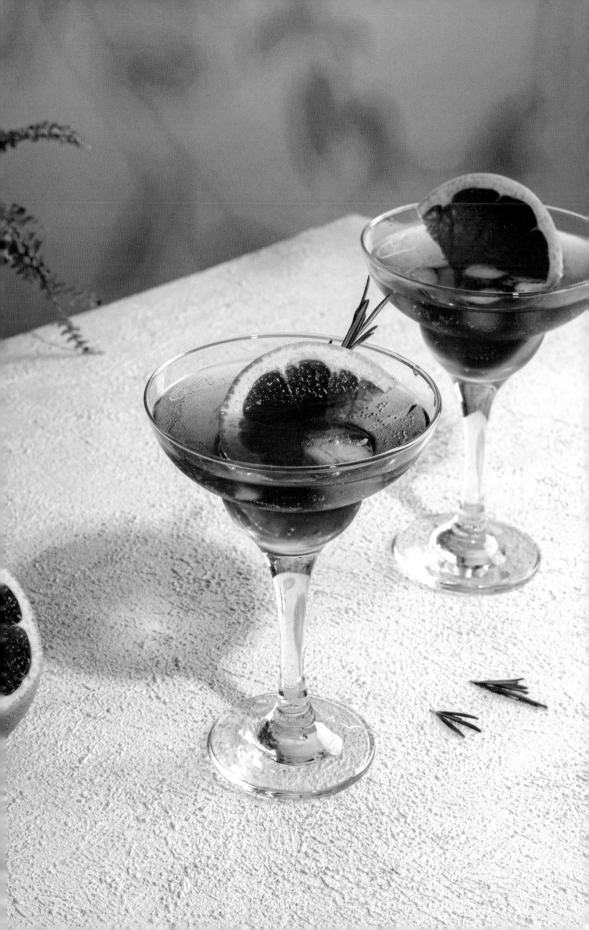

# Index

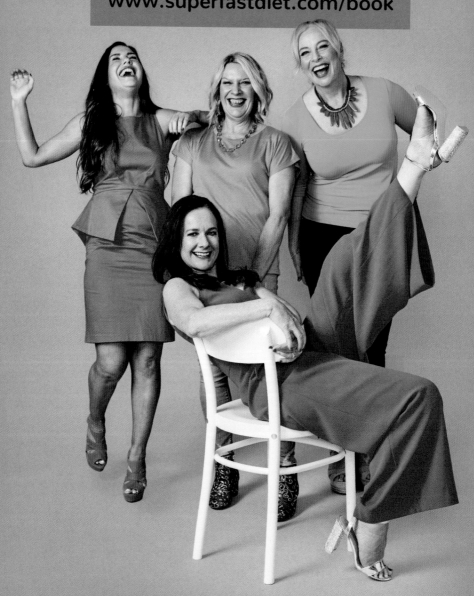

## OUR ONLINE PROGRAM INCLUDES:

- STACKS more recipes, sample days, meal plans and snack options
- Your very own dashboard, tracker and vision board
- Exclusive access to our SUPER community

- Super-motivating twice-weekly coaching videos from our celebrity supporters and world-leading experts
- A specially designed DOABLE exercise series
- A super-mindset series

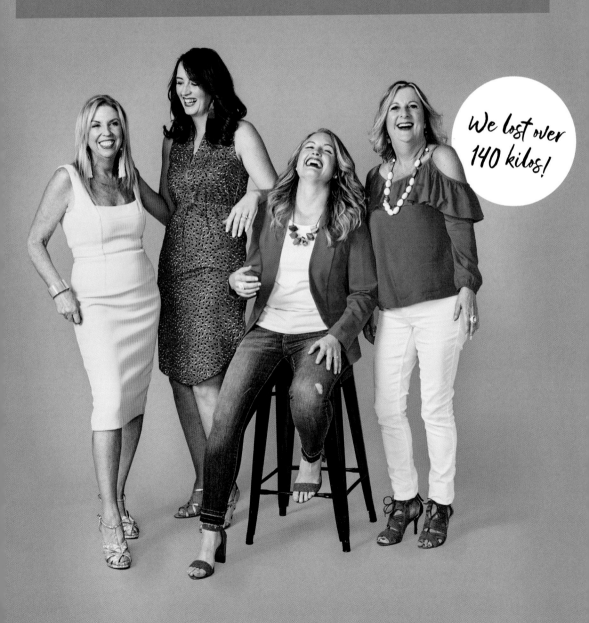

We lost over 140 kilos!

Pan Macmillan acknowledges the Traditional Custodians of Country throughout Australia and their connections to lands, waters and communities. We pay our respect to Elders past and present and extend that respect to all Aboriginal and Torres Strait Islander peoples today. We honour more than sixty thousand years of storytelling, art and culture.

First published 2023 in Australia
by Pan Macmillan Australia Pty Limited
Level 25, 1 Market Street, Sydney, New South Wales
Australia 2000

Text copyright © Victoria Black and Gen Davidson 2023
Photography Rob Palmer and Jeremy Simons copyright © Pan Macmillan 2023

Image on pages 4–5, 9, 20, 26–27, 30, 42–43, 50, 66, 78, 104, 107, 110, 111, and 230–231 © Shutterstock; image on pages 6–7, 20, 28–29, 34, 35, 39, 46, 63, 66, 78, 79, 84, 88-89, 90, 106, 240 and 93, 233 © iStock.

 A catalogue record for this book is available from the National Library of Australia
NATIONAL LIBRARY OF AUSTRALIA

Design by Madeleine Kane
Recipe development by Meg Yonson
Edited by Ariana Klepac
Index by Jenny Browne
Prop and food styling by Vanessa Austin and Emma Knowles

Food preparation by Kerrie Ray
Colour + reproduction by Splitting Image Colour Studio
Printed in China by Imago Printing International Limited

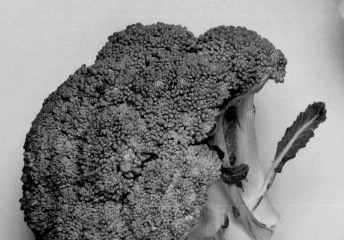